ALCOHOLISM AND WOMEN, GENETICS, AND FETAL DEVELOPMENT

The Six Volumes in This Series Are:

1. *Alcoholism: Its Natural History, Chemistry and General Metabolism*
2. *The Neurobiology of Alcohol Abuse*
3. *The Psychodynamics of Alcoholism: A Current Synthesis*
4. *Alcoholism and Women, Genetics, and Fetal Development*
5. *Alcoholism and Polydrug Abuse, Co-Dependency, Recovery, and the Role of the Clinician*
6. *The Pharmacology of Drugs Other than Alcohol*

ALCOHOLISM AND WOMEN, GENETICS, AND FETAL DEVELOPMENT

By

WILLIAM J. HAUGEN LIGHT, PH.D.

Institute for the Study of Drugs,
Alcohol, and Addictive Behaviors
and
Department of Biology
Metropolitan State College
Denver, Colorado
Research Associate
California Academy of Sciences

CHARLES C THOMAS • PUBLISHER
Springfield • Illinois • U. S. A.

Published and Distributed Throughout the World by

CHARLES C THOMAS • PUBLISHER
2600 South First Street
Springfield, Illinois 62794-9265

ISBN 0-398-05399-5

Library of Congress Catalog Card Number: 87-18031

With THOMAS BOOKS *careful attention is given to all details of manufacturing and design. It is the Publisher's desire to present books that are satisfactory as to their physical qualities and artistic possibilities and appropriate for their particular use.* THOMAS BOOKS *will be true to those laws of quality that assure a good name and good will.*

Printed in the United States of America
Q-R-3

Library of Congress Cataloging in Publication Data

Light, William J. Haugen.
Alcoholism and women, genetics, and fetal development.

Constitutes v. 4 of an untitled series.
Bibliography: p.
Includes index.
1. Alcoholism—Genetic aspects. 2. Women—Alcohol use. 3. Fetal alcohol syndrome. I. Title. [DNLM: 1. Alcoholism. 2. Alcoholism—familial & genetic. 3. Fetal Alcohol Syndrome. WM 274 L723a]
RC565.L538 1988 616.86'1 87-18031
ISBN 0-398-05399-5

TO THE MEMORY of my brother-friend, James Buffington Jordan, who departed this life so unexpectedly: for afternoons on the Upper Duck and discussions of the Gateless Gate deep into the night—but most of all for a lifetime of companionship and sharing. My wife, our two daughters and I miss him enormously.

PREFACE

THIS SERIES of volumes is written as an introduction to the complex and often bewildering illness of alcoholism. It is directed primarily to health care professionals, particularly medical students, practicing physicians, psychiatric and psychological clinicians and trainees, nurses, alcoholism counselors, and other practitioners who regularly confront alcoholism as either the primary illness or as a major complicating factor in their patients or clients. One may legitimately ask, why another series on alcoholism? They seem to be coming off the presses at a brisk rate already from nearly every quarter—as though another new fad has burst upon us and one is not really "with it" unless one is either a recovered alcoholic intent upon telling his or her own story, or else is involved in treating them in some way. One can scarcely keep up with the literature in one's own specialty, let alone the proliferation of books and articles about alcoholism. Why burden us with yet more?

My response is that the works currently available overwhelmingly treat the subject from the fairly narrow perspective in which the authors or editors are themselves research experts, or out of the need to advance a favorite model or theory about the cause(s), course and preferred treatment of the problem. Or if they are more general and ecclectic in scope, the discussion is far too superficial to be of any real value for professional workers who wish to know the current state of our knowledge of "ethanology." The last ten years or so have seen an enormous growth in our understanding about alcohol and alcoholism research. At some point in the very recent past we acquired a critical mass of accurate, scientific information about the pharmacological mechanisms by which alcohol (and many other addictive agents, as well) affects membrane systems and leads to pharmacological tolerance and physical dependence. These data, coupled with an increasingly sophisticated understanding of the psychodynamic and biochemical factors contributing to psychiatric illness in general and our ability to effectively intervene in such illnesses to an unprecedented degree, have permitted an understanding of alcoholic disorders at a most fundamental level—a level that rivals our comprehension of our world and our universe in the other cognate sciences.

This information, unfortunately, is widely scattered in numerous professional journals and symposium volumes in the fields of medicine, toxicology and pharmacology, physiology, psychiatry and psychology. It is also heavily burdened with highly technical jargon and it assumes a command of the relevant background literature that is rarely possessed by anyone not actively working in the research frontiers of the respective discipline. These comments also apply to recent reviews on the subject (for example, Lieber 1982).

It was my intention to bring together the substance of this vast literature, organize it into what I hope is a holistic and coherent picture, and translate it into comprehensible English that can be readily understood by any reasonably intelligent and educated person. I am convinced that this can be accomplished without sacrificing any of the scientific accuracy or subtle nuances of understanding to be obtained from close attention to the fine details and interrelationships of the various systems involved.

Thus, an adequate comprehension of the many factors contributing to alcoholic liver disease requires a detailed knowledge of liver structure and function. It is especially important to know how the structural units of the liver typically described in medical texts correlate with the physiologically more useful "functional" hepatic units, the liver acini, and how their concentric zones of increasing anoxia toward the perivenular areas lead to specific regional hepatic lesions, necrosis, and ultimately, fibrosis. One must also be aware of the biochemical details of the mixed-function monooxygenases, basic pharmacokinetics and enzymatic processes, general lipid metabolism, the involvement of the pituitary-adrenal axis and catecholamine release upon peripheral free fatty acid mobilization, and the bewildering array of metabolic consequences of altered redox states resulting from alcohol oxidation.

This series is meant to be a current synthesis of information from many different fields and an examination of the disease of alcoholism as I have come to know it over nearly 18 years of professional study. It is based, among other things, upon my experience in working with alcoholics and their families as supervising counselor for the National Council on Alcoholism in the San Francisco Bay area. It incorporates a background and education spanning many years as a professional scientist and educator and which includes formal training in toxicology at the University of Wisconsin at Madison. It grew out of a series of lectures that I developed for a wide range of audiences, ranging from youngsters on probation for alcohol and drug related offenses, through volunteer workers and counselor-trainees in alcohol intervention, to formal classes of nursing and medical students at the University of San Francisco and the University of California School of Medicine at San Francisco, and finally, both undergraduate and graduate level courses in pharmacology of addictions at Metropolitan State College and the University of Colorado, both schools in Denver.

Although I have assumed no particular background or professional training on the part of the readers it is expected that they have at least some basic understanding of the nature of chemical bonds and can comprehend the simple structural formulae presented herein. Those with absolutely no understanding of these concepts are referred to the chapters on the chemistry of life to be found in any good biology textbook. These subjects are also discussed more fully in the first volume of this series (Light 1985).

Some readers will perhaps have psychological foundations, some medical, some may be members of the clergy, some paraprofessional counselors of various persuasions with or without formal scientific training, and some may be interested laypersons who are themselves recovering or recovered alcoholics or the close friends and significant others of alcoholics. Because of the disparate backgrounds of the readership to which this series of books is directed, I have introduced each topic with a basic examination of the terminology and processes under discussion. The reader is led step by step through ever more advanced and sophisticated concepts up to and including the latest information, ideas, and thinking entertained by current researchers in the field.

Therefore, a family practice or general physician may be initially annoyed at elementary discussions of such things as oxidation-reduction reactions. These are included, however, so that someone from another discipline, let us say clinical psychology, will be able to follow subsequent treatments of the metabolic significance of altered redox states consequent to the oxidation of large amounts of alcohol and the ultimate effects of these processes upon human cognition and behavior.

The medically or biologically sophisticated reader will soon enough encounter very detailed presentations of biochemical phenomena that are currently at the forefronts of scientific investigation—subjects that will most certainly not have been studied if he or she has been in practice for even a very few years (like less than five or six). Indeed, many of these subjects have yet to be incorporated into standard medical texts or curricula. At the same time, our clinical psychologist will have been educated up to the level of the medical or research professional, at least insofar as is immediately relevant to a full understanding of the topic under consideration. Elsewhere the situation will be reversed, so that it is now the psychiatrically erudite reader who must tolerate the initial, elementary presentation of such things as depressive-spectrum disorder, sociopathy and its relationship to primary and secondary alcoholism and the rudimentary concepts of decompensation and regression, narcissistic trauma and entitlement loss. But here, too, the discussion will soon lead into such topics as the interrelationship between narcissism and paranoid ideation in alcoholics, dyadic versus triadic conflicts, and the relative degrees of bonding and socialization in the development of the psychoses, neuroses and personality disorders. The latest concepts involving imbalances of central neurotransmitter substances as major factors in psychiatric disturbances, including alcoholism, are explored in depth and fully integrated with more traditional psychodynamic models. I believe this series represents the only work to date that truly accomplishes this goal in a fundamental and coherent way.

I am introducing a number of ideas of my own about alcoholism which are presented for the first time in this series of volumes. I do have personal biases about this disorder, as does anyone who has thought about it seriously for more than ten minutes. Some of these ideas conflict with certain theories of some other authors. This is most evident in the portions dealing with the etiological factors underlying alcoholism, a subject which has spawned much often acrimonious debate. However, my suggestions are quite in line with the medical and psychiatric consensus about alcoholic disorders, and they are thoughts to which I have given careful consideration and brought wide-ranging knowledge and experience. I cannot prove some of these ideas, but I think they are as valid as anyone's. They are based upon personal insight and understanding, both intuitive and scientifically objective, of the various dynamics involved. They are certainly no more flimsily grounded than is most of the clinical and psychiatric literature, which is similarly anecdotal. The major portion of this work is, of course, firmly based upon solidly demonstrated, scientific data—particularly those sections dealing with the pharmacological and biological aspects of alcoholism.

Although much of the material contained in these volumes is difficult and complex, it is presented in what I hope is an easy, communicative, and readable style. I have provided a great many graphic illustrations to aid the users of these books, and innumerable footnotes supply additional information to enhance a point or to correlate the discussion with other related phenomena. I have not encumbered the text with extensive citations from the professional literature. This information is in the public domain and is well documented by the references which I do include. This series is also not intended to be an exhaustive, encyclopaedic catalog of facts and statistics about alcoholism. Rather, it attempts to provide a comprehensive and holistic synthesis of the many interrelated psychodynamic and biological processes which contribute to the etiology and manifestations of alcoholic disorders. The information contained herein is the product of a huge army of investigators and clinicians in many fields whose work spans many decades. I have served primarily as an interpreter.

I have covered little of the ground previously discussed for general audiences by other authors, although some review of such information is appropriate and is included. An example is a detailed presentation of the course of primary alcoholism as originally described by the late Dr. E. M. Jellinek. But even here, the discussion has been modernized and tempered with a much wider clinical experience than was available in Jellinek's time. And a few qualifying remarks of my own are included. I will not go very deeply into the various debates on treatment modalities, although I will present a broad approach based upon the overwhelming medical and psychiatric consensus in the final volume of this series. And I do not propose to engage in the endless debate about whether alcoholics can safely return to drinking on a social basis. I will categorically state my firm conviction that they cannot, and that any attempt to suggest that they can is medically and psychiatrically irresponsible. As to the sections dealing with the pharmacology, toxicology and metabolism of alcohol, and the genetics, biology, natural history and medical aspects of alcoholism, my discussions are confined to hard, scientifically verifiable facts and interpretations, and any inferences I may draw are based upon these hard data and are also supported in the professional literature.

I had originally intended to write a book for the recovering alcoholic and his or her family, inasmuch as many of them, regardless of the particular treatment modality in which they may be participating, are largely ignorant about the disease, its causes, course, and medical and psychological consequences (as are the great majority of health care professionals).

Although many alcoholics make full recoveries and are able to lead rich and satisfying lives, many others are plagued by recurrent or chronic depressions of profound proportions and are afflicted by a variety of physical and emotional problems that require professional intervention—a form of assistance they all too rarely get.

But as the manuscript progressed it became apparent that I was getting far too deep into the scientific details and complexities of the alcoholic disorders to keep the attention of most laypersons for long. This was obviously the case despite my efforts to make it palatable to a wide range of readers and clearly understandable by any fairly intelligent and literate person willing to put in the necessary effort. About this time my wife, who is a practicing physician, suggested that I was actually writing for a professional audience and that I should continue in that genre. She observed that a much less detailed synopsis of this work would be more appropriate for the average reader.

What I have done in this series is to provide a thorough and detailed introduction into each discipline so that nonspecialists will understand the many intricacies of normal function of each system under consideration. Thus, the volume dealing with the effects of alcohol and alcoholism upon the human nervous system begins with a review of basic neurobiology. One has to know how neurons function and transmit information before one can appreciate how alcohol affects those processes. Similarly, one cannot really appreciate the ways in which alcohol ravages embryonic development or understand fetal alcohol syndrome without some basic knowledge of normal human fetal development. So each topic is presented as a detailed minicourse for those who know little or nothing about it. This is true of the psychodynamics volumes as well as the biologically and medically oriented ones. Following the introductory sections, the effects of alcohol and alcohol abuse upon the respective systems are presented in great detail. In this book, certain basic ideas in genetics and the development of the central nervous system are presented in appendices one and two. Certain fundamental biochemical and neurobiological concepts discussed in volumes 1 and 2 of this series (Light 1985 and 1986a, respectively) are not repeated in the later volumes, and the reader is referred to those volumes if clarification is required. And similarly, the psychological factors underlying alcoholism are explored in depth in volume 3 (Light 1986b).

This series of volumes presents, I believe, as complete an integrated a picture of alcoholism as it is currently possible to create. And I think the model described in this series is a powerful and useful one. Alcoholism, perhaps more than most psychiatric disorders, can be understood at several fundamental levels. This series of books is my contribution to that end.

This work took four years to complete, and the final manuscript was more than 1,000 pages and a quarter of a million words in length. There were some 90 full page illustrations. Because of the enormous cost of producing a single or even two-volume book from this manuscript, costs which would have priced this work far beyond the reach of most of us (including myself), the publisher and I agreed to present this as a series of six volumes, each about 200 or so pages long. To fully grasp the entire picture requires all six of these volumes. Nevertheless, each one is self-contained and presents a complete picture of alcoholism and the respective topics contained therein.

I, at least, have grown enormously both professionally and personally by writing this series. It has enabled me to provide my students at the Institute for the Study of Drugs, Alcohol and Addictive Behaviors at Metropolitan State College and the University of Colorado at Denver with extraordinarily valuable information and insight to take with them into the world of addiction prevention, intervention, treatment, and education.

W.J.H.L.

Colorado Springs

ACKNOWLEDGMENTS

I OWE AN enormous debt to many individuals, organizations and institutions who made this series possible. Among these are: Mrs. Florette White Pomeroy, retired executive director of the National Council on Alcoholism—Bay Area, who gave me free rein during my tenure there and staunchly supported my sometimes unusual methods of intervention; Dr. Mary Fortin, formerly of the School of Nursing at the University of San Francsico; Dr. Mark I. Levy, a loyal companion in a common cause who walked an enormous distance with me along the incredible path of discovery and enlightenment; Dr. Antonio J. Ferreira, who freely shared many of his keen insights with me deriving from his private psychiatric practice focusing on alcoholics and their families; Mr. Mitch Capor of the Alameda County Probation Department, California, who provided an ongoing opportunity to gain valuable insight into the special problems of teenage substance abuse; my wife, Dr. Ruth Lewert Light, who has been a constant source of strength and inspiration throughout both our lives together and the writing of this manuscript; and my students in introductory and advanced courses in pharmacology and psychodynamics of addictions at the Institute for the Study of Drugs, Alcohol, and Addictive Behaviors at both Metropolitan State College and the University of Colorado at Denver, who force me to continually consolidate, sharpen and refine my thoughts about the subject and who always remind me of my vast ignorance.

Words cannot express my deep gratitude to the many thousands of men and women in Alcoholics Anonymous and its sister fellowship, Al-Anon. Perhaps this series of volumes may be regarded as a small repayment for all the pain and joy that they have shared with me and for the many lifetime friendships that have sprung up between us. This work is for them, the recovered and recovering alcoholics and co-alcoholics, who have shown the way to so many thousands of suffering victims of this most horrible of afflictions.

I also thank Payne Thomas and his staff at Charles C Thomas, Publisher for their kind cooperation and for the speed and skill with which they have processed these six manuscripts. It is a privilege and a pleasure to have worked with them. Paul Schoen of Keyser Litho, Inc. in Colorado Springs, skillfully made the many plates and figures into fine, camera-ready prints, and Cindy Sorensen carefully and accurately typed the final manuscripts.

Dr. George Henry and David Peakman of the Cytogenetics Laboratory, Reproductive Genetics Center, Denver, Colorado, kindly provided the karyotype of the author's youngest daughter (Figure 3).

Finally, I thank Drs. John J. Magnuson and Ronald D. Hinsdill of the University of Wisconsin at Madison, who provided more than they know, who good naturedly tolerated my eccentricities, and who generously allowed me to wear both my hats simultaneously.

The writing of this manuscript was supported in part by the Department of Health and Human Services Public Health Service National Research Award 5 T32 ES05015 to the University of Wisconsin from the National Institute of Environmental Health Sciences.

LIST OF FIGURES

CONTENTS

ALCOHOLISM AND WOMEN, GENETICS, AND FETAL DEVELOPMENT

AN INTRODUCTORY NOTE

THIS CHAPTER on alcoholism and women attempts only to present the preponderance of the findings of studies dealing with this subject. Despite numerous methodological, sociological, and "feminist" criticism of this literature, there does seem to be a general agreement about most of these findings. Throughout this work I have not engaged in, and do not propose to do so, any debate about feminist or other current ideological issues for several reasons: (1) I do not understand most of these issues and I have little to say about them; (2) I do not believe that most of them are really relevant to the perspective presented here; and (3) there is at present no reasonable way of even approximately testing the validity of such claims and counterclaims. Thus, the recent emancipation of American women with its associated benefits and problems for both sexes is not really discussed with respect to its impact upon alcoholism in women. Although this sociological phenomenon has many wide-ranging and important consequences for us all, its role in the etiology and manifestations of female alcoholism is not at all understood, even by those who claim otherwise. My intention in this book is to present an organic natural history of the disorder based upon innate physiological, biochemical, and psychodynamic substrates and stresses. To the extent that sociological and demographic factors are known to be involved, that material has been briefly discussed in the introductory chapter of the first volume of this series (Light 1985). These approaches have been more than adequately treated in numerous other works and the reader is referred there for further enlightenment (for example, MacLennan 1976; Tarter and Sugarman 1976; Burtle 1980; Camberwell Council on Alcoholism 1980; Corrigan 1980; Galanter 1980; Sandmaier 1980). As important as these issues are and despite the enrichment they bring to the subject, I do not think that they would alter the themes presented here in any fundamental way given their current state of disciplinary development.

Although I agree with those critics who charge that Freud was himself a shameless male chauvinist who considered women to be biologically and psychologically inferior to man (however, one must consider the times, in his defense), I do not believe that all of psychoanalytic theory should be thrown out with the wash water (see for example, Saunders 1980). Just because one is upset with the personality foibles of the formulator of a model that offers a great deal of valuable insight is no valid ground for rejecting the whole bag of apples. Despite its many shortcomings and the real advances in our understanding of human behavior represented by several recent psychodynamic models, psychoanalytic theory is still very much a meaningful, relevant and enlightening approach to understanding how people think, feel and behave. Newtonian physics was by no means invalidated by quantum mechanics, but rather restricted to the special case of phenomena in the macroscopic world—we still build our bridges and direct our space satellites by Newtonian mechanics, after all. Similarly, psychoanalytic theory as it is currently understood remains our most useful *single* model with regard to human psychodynamics. When combined with modern psychopharmacology and biochemistry (Freud, after all, was firmly convinced of the fundamental biological basis of all psychiatric disturbance), our comprehension of and ability to effectively intervene in mental disorders is powerful indeed—and appears highly likely to become even more so in the near future.

All psychological models are ultimately based upon personal insight and intuition, including those deriving from batteries of statistical testing protocols—the tests, after all, were themselves developed from the authors' own insights and hunches about what qualities are likely to be associated with which psychological sets and modes. I hope my more activist-minded readers will forgive this self-imposed restriction in my discussion of this disorder; they are certainly free to pursue those lines of inquiry on their own. My book is based upon those factors that I believe I understand well enough to coherently integrate and present in one major work.

ALCOHOLISM IN WOMEN

ALTHOUGH the literature on alcoholism in women has been meagre, such studies have been appearing at an increasing rate in recent years (for example, Lisansky 1957, 1960; Kinsey 1966; Gomberg 1976; Burtle 1979; Fine *et al.*, Morrissey and Schuckit, and Richman *et al., in*: Galanter 1980). With some qualifications they generally agree that alcoholism as it is expressed in women differs significantly from that seen in men in the following ways:

(1) Women generally begin to drink pathologically at a later age than do men; unlike men, who gradually slide into alcoholic drinking over a prolonged period, women are much more likely to associate one or more specific traumatic events with the rapid onset of alcoholic drinking.

(2) Despite the onset of alcoholic drinking at a later age, women typically show a "telescoped," more rapid progression of their alcoholism, and they are first hospitalized for medical complications of chronic alcohol abuse at about the same age as men.

(3) For obscure reasons they are more prone to develop alcoholic liver cirrhosis than men and they die from the medical consequences of their alcoholism at a younger age than do men; liver cirrhosis is twice as common among women than it is among men even though they generally drink less long and consume less alcohol per day than men.

(4) Alcoholism among women is generally associated with greater psychopathology, especially major depression, than it is in men, and women are much more likely to have a previous history of psychiatric treatment (but see qualifying comments below).

(5) Women are much more likely than men to be polydrug abusers, particularly with regard to prescribed and over the counter medications; this may reflect the fact that women in the general populations tend to make greater use of medications than do men.

(6) Female alcoholics are less likely than males to drink every day or to "binge" drink; they are more likely to drink alone or to drink with a

spouse or male companion, perhaps reflecting their traditional roles as housewives and the greater social condemnation directed towards alcoholism in women.

(7) Women are less likely to be arrested for alcohol-related offenses or to lose their jobs due to alcoholism (this last at least partly reflecting the fact that fewer women than men occupy jobs).

(8) Female alcoholics are much more likely than males to have married one or more times and their marriages are typically much more dysfunctional than those of male alcoholics—women are much more frequently divorced than their male counterparts.

The initiation of drinking by previously teetotalling individuals, particularly women, in later life associated with an exceptionally rapid progression of florid alcoholism has been mentioned in the introductory volume of this series (Light 1985). This may be related to the strange phenomenon of alcoholic progression that seems to occur even in abstinent alcoholics, resulting in the almost immediate or at least rapid manifestation of much more severe signs of alcoholic deterioration upon resumption of drinking than were present when the alcoholic became abstinent. On the other hand, it may well represent an extreme variant of the general tendency for a more rapid progression of alcoholism among women, and the fact that the onset of alcoholism in this group is typically associated with one or more specific and traumatic precipitating life events. This telescoped progression is characteristic of the lone female alcoholic who begins to drink at a later age than the mean for all female alcoholics. Among those alcoholic women who begin drinking at an early age, the progression is much less rapid and less dramatic (Kinsey 1966).

Whereas the majority of male alcoholics are diagnosed as having primary alcoholism (the situation in sociopathic male alcoholics being unclear), there is nearly universal agreement that alcoholism in women is secondary to an underlying affective disorder—*viz.*, major depression (Burns 1979). However, alcoholism among males is also generally accompanied by major depression, and despite some claims to the contrary (for example, Vaillant 1983), this depression far more often than not precedes the onset of alcoholic drinking, and is usually present in childhood. Alcoholism-associated depression among males is generally not as clinically obvious as it is in women, and males are much more likely to exhibit agitated features than are women, whose depression is much more likely to show psychomotor retardation. Male alcoholics generally resemble the symptomatic cluster associated with "reactive" or "neurotic" depression, whereas women usually present a symptomatology that fits the criteria for "endogenous" or "psychotic" depression.

Depression is closely associated with alcoholism in both males and females. Females from families in which alcoholism is present are more likely than males to develop a primary depressive disorder, whereas the males from such families more frequently develop alcoholism or sociopathy. This family picture fits the definition of *depressive spectrum disorder* and any depressive illness in such a family is appropriately given that diagnosis (see also Winokur 1979; Light 1986b). It has been repeatedly emphasized in this series that the entire range of depressive disorders[1] probably represents a phenotypic continuum with an underlying polygenic basis. Females in the general population are more often diagnosed as having a primary affective disturbance than are men, and depression in women more often exhibits the so-called "vegetative" symptomatic picture generally associated with endogenous depression. Major depression very often occurs in the absence of any accompanying alcoholism, but alcoholism is almost never found in the absence of a moderate to severe clinical depression. As previously mentioned, alcoholism does indeed feed into and greatly exacerbate any co-existing depression, so that the clinical picture presented by both male and female advanced alcoholics is a composite one including factors which represent both cause and effect of long-term, chronic alcohol abuse. Alcoholism is both genetically and psychodynamically intertwined with the affective disorders, and it is my contention that alcoholics of both sexes represent a sub-category of affective illness—especially of depression.[2]

Most studies agree that women alcoholics exhibit greater psychopathology and social deviancy than do men, but the extent to which societal norms and expectations regarding alcoholism in women contribute to this judgment is by no means clear. The very fact that a woman *is* an alcoholic carries with it a much greater social stigma than is true in the case of male alcoholics. Much of the negative response towards female alcoholism derives from deep-seated feelings society has about the projected indifference of female drunkards towards spouse and children,

---

[1]All psychiatric disturbances are accompanied by at least some symptoms of depression. In the context of this work depression is restricted to those disorders in which the major presenting picture fits the formal criteria of the affective disorders. The close relationship between the various types of depression is reflected in DSM-III, which places them all into a single major diagnostic category.

[2]Bipolar disorder is also sometimes seen in alcoholic patients, but the relationship here is far more obscure and even the alcoholic picture is sometimes atypical.

and fears of their promiscuous sexual acting-out while drunk.[3] Being so stigmatized as automatically more "deviant" carries its own self-fulfilling prophesy: women are labelled more deviant, therefore they *are* more deviant. And such labelling inevitably feeds into and worsens their already negative self-image, which in itself can hardly avoid disrupting already weak ego-strengths and generating further demoralization and psychopathology. It is possible that only more deviant women would ever slip into alcoholic drinking given the strong social opprobrium against female drunkenness, but this argument is not very convincing. *No one* ever sets out to become an alcoholic! Alcoholism in both men and women is a deadly, insidious and progressive malady that sneaks up on its victims and totally ensnares them before they can realize what is happening to them. By the time they are caught it is far too late to stop the onslaught, short of hitting their individual "bottom" and entering a successful treatment program. All the above said, it does appear that both practicing and recovering women alcoholics more often suffer from an often severe and debilitating, endogenous-type depression. Male alcoholics more often present an often intense, anxious and "agitated" type of depression which is generally not as clinically obvious, but which is largely responsible for the irritability and chronic state of anger, frequent temper outbursts, and low tolerance to frustration commonly seen in this group. These features are present in both practicing and abstinent alcoholics, but they tend to be most pronounced for a varying period of time following abstinence from alcohol.[4]

That female alcoholics much more frequently abuse drugs other than alcohol gives support to the idea that they are psychiatrically more disturbed than males. They are more prone to suicide attempts, acts that are facilitated by the compounding of their depression by multiple sedative-hypnotic agents like alcohol, barbiturates and benzodiazepines which act in concert to potentiate central depression (in both senses of that word). There is a general correlation between psychosocial

[3]There is no evidence that female alcoholics are any more promiscuous or engage in more sexual acting-out than non-alcoholic women, except perhaps in the case of some lower-class, inner-city women or those with sociopathic features.

[4]Except in far-advanced, chronic alcoholism, ethanol serves as an effective anti-depressant "medication," perhaps especially in cases of serotonin dysfunction and the presumably resulting agitated type of depression (see Light 1986a). Alcohol thus blocks most of the symptoms that derive from such depression. Upon prolonged abstinence the depressive symptoms tend to emerge fullblown and unchecked, and they may even be worsened because of the rebound effect of serotoninergic neuroreceptors. Such symptoms are very common in abstinent, recovering alcoholics, often for a period of several years or more, and they are often referred to as "dry drunks" by members of Alcoholics Anonymous.

deviancy and the use of a wider variety of drugs for non-therapeutic purposes.[5]

However, women in this society much more frequently take a wide variety of both over the counter and prescription medications for legitimate purposes. The polydrug abuse so prevalent among female alcohol abusers, therefore, may merely be an extension of their normal penchant for wide use of medications. As such, it may not represent any greater psychopathology than is found among men, simply because such drug use is in fact not deviant and lies well within normal limits for American women. Once uncontrolled and compulsive overindulgence in one drug (alcohol) is established it automatically includes other addiction-prone chemicals, and a vicious cycle of polydrug abuse is kindled. Because the combined effects of polydrug abuse are much more disruptive than are those of alcoholism alone, a much more severe psychopathology almost inevitably ensues which may well be reflected in the clinically greater psychiatric disturbance seen in alcoholic women.

The fact that alcoholic women more often have a history of psychiatric treatment may be due to a greater incidence of psychopathology relative to their male counterparts. However, it may also reflect a greater reluctance by women to acknowledge their alcoholism and to seek other causes for their distressed and chaotic lives. Their physicians are likewise very prone to go into collusion with this fiction, diagnosing them as "psychoneurotic" or "hysterical"—both much more socially acceptable disorders—and refer them for psychiatric treatment. There is still a very strong tendency for health care professionals to regard alcohol abuse as being symptomatic of underlying psychological difficulties. Although psychiatric distress always accompanies alcoholism and at least depression usually exists prior to the onset of pathological drinking, the one most effective and important endeavor the physician can undertake is to recognize alcoholism as the primary illness that it is (depression being merely one component) and to direct his main interventive efforts toward attaining and maintaining complete and permanent abstinence. Without effectively interdicting the alcoholism, there is no hope of ameliorating other co-occurring medical and/or psychiatric problems.

[5]By "non-therapeutic" I also mean the excessive misuse of prescribed medications intended for moderate use to alleviate anxiety and tension. The use of any drug or medication other than exactly as prescribed constitutes drug misuse. And the responsibility for that misuse and its consequences fall squarely on the patient.

A recent study by Morrissey and Schuckit (1980) shows that lower-class alcoholic women closely resemble their middle-class counterparts in most details. Although the proportions of specific problems relative to lower-class males are about the same as in middle-class populations, lower-class women show an earlier age of first occurrences for these problems. They are as likely as their male counterparts to have a history of juvenile delinquency and detention and nearly as likely to engage in physical fights and to use a weapon with intent to injure their opponent. They are more likely to have borne children than males are to have fathered offspring, and they are much more likely to be living with others. Lower-class male alcoholics experience all kinds of psychosocial and medical problems much more frequently than their female counterparts, except for withdrawal tremors and diagnosed liver damage in which the ratios were sharply reversed.

Despite the foregoing differences in drinking patterns and behavior between men and women alcoholics, the two sexes appear to be psychologically more alike than non-alike (Gomberg 1976). The fundamental psychodynamic factors do not seem to differ significantly between male and female alcoholics whether these two groups are assessed clinically (intuitively) or by means of psychological tests such as the Minnesota Multiphasic Personality Inventory (MMPI). One study (Mogar *et al.*, 1970, *in:* Gomberg 1976) reported five distinct MMPI profiles among female alcoholics: normal, depressive, "hysterical," psychopathic, and passive-aggressive; and four types among men: passive-aggressive, depressive-compulsive, "schizoid prepsychotic," and passive-dependent. Others (Hoffmann and Jackson 1974, *ibid.*) show that male alcoholics score significantly higher in character disorder traits and female alcoholics to have significantly more neurotic features.

There is consistent agreement that female alcoholics deviate further from normal feminine behavior than alcoholic males do from normal male behavior (Gomberg 1976). Such deviancy should not, however, be taken to necessarily mean that female alcoholics are more pathological than male alcoholics. It does imply that women alcohol abusers suffer at least to some degree more severe sanctions from society, which would seem almost surely to exaggerate their negative self-images, depression and demoralization, and feelings of remorse, self-loathing and uncertainty. The proportion of successful interventions in female alcoholism does not appear to be significantly lower than it is in males, although this might be expected if there were a greater pathology among the former (Kinsey 1966).

Sex role issues constitute major problems for both male and female alcoholics. Female alcoholics tend to emphasize and value traditional feminine behavior traits and activities, whereas alcoholic men similarly overemphasize traditional masculine behaviors and activities. However, nearly all investigators agree that such role overemphasis constitutes an overdetermined reaction formation to fundamental conflicts about sex roles and their own identity as males or females. Ambiguity and ambivalence dominate the alcoholic's relationship to practically *everything* in both men and women. Despite such confusion about identity and sexual roles "latent homosexuality" is no more an etiological factor in alcoholism in women than it is in men (Kinsey 1966).

The few studies to date concerning the psychodynamic factors associated with alcoholism in women paint a remarkably similar picture to that seen among male alcoholics. Despite minor disagreements in the literature, the following features are frequently reported (Kinsey 1966; Gomberg 1976; Jacobson 1980):

(1) A high frequency of traumatic early life experiences including loss of a parent, active alcoholism and/or other psychiatric illness in the family, rejection and other stressful factors which interfere with the child's ability to form healthy interpersonal relationships, thus leading to isolation and loneliness.

(2) An unusually ambivalent relationship to the father who was typically alcoholic, psychotic or absent from home (or when he was home there was severe family conflict), coupled with hostility toward the mother. Both boys and girls tend to respond to frightening and dangerous family acting-out patterns with the primitive ego-defense mechanism known as *splitting* (see Light 1986b).[6] This can lead to depersonalization and emotional shallowness, and to schizoid, avoidant and borderline personality traits.

(3) As already discussed, identity and sex role confusion often lead

[6]Splitting is the response of the primitive, pre-Oedipal ego to frustrating or rejecting object experiences. Good or satisfying object experiences (for example, times when the alcoholic parent is sober and loving) are totally introjected and bad or unsatisfying experiences are totally projected and maintained separately. This rigid separation is maintained in order to avoid the intense anxiety associated with ambivalence—that is, the presence of both good and bad elements in the same person. Persistent splitting leads to reaction formation, repression and denial, an impaired and immature ego incapable of accommodating contrasting features in the same object—thus causing dysfunctional interpersonal relationships, and an extremely low tolerance for anxiety, ambivalence and ambiguity.

to overemphasis of feminine traits, including passive-submissive social and interpersonal behavior.[7]

(4) Strong feelings of self-depreciation and intense feelings of inferiority and insecurity together with deep needs and strivings for love and acceptance by others are prominent features of alcoholism in women; such women are forever striving for love and appreciation while simultaneously suffering intense fear of rejection and rebuff. Despite their desperate need for intimacy and human contact, they, like their male counterparts, typically stagger through one pathological relationship after another or remain continuously isolated and alone.

(5) Psychosexual development remains largely fixated at the oral stage and the personality is dominated by dependency and passivity, despite counterdependent behavior by some women; there is inadequate tolerance for frustration, delay, and they are easily disappointed and largely unable to control their impulses.

(6) Like their male counterparts, female alcoholics experience great difficulty making adjustments to adult roles and responsibilities, resulting in still further confusion in self-image and identity and precipitating a global retreat behind a defensive facade. This protective bulwark represents a "shotgun-strategy" hodgepodge of aggressiveness, superficial self-confidence and independence, defiance, hostility, and self-hatred (Kinsey 1966) underlain by poorly repressed and overwhelming feelings of inadequacy and self-loathing.

Alcoholics constitute a more heterogeneous population than are typical for other psychiatric disorders, and there is general agreement in the literature that alcoholics do not fall into any one single personality profile. Nevertheless, the consensus also exists that depression and psychopathy (sociopathy) are strongly linked to alcoholism and that both appear to be clear predisposing factors in its etiology. It is also clear that females from families with alcoholism, psychopathy or depression are more likely to present with clinical depression, whereas males from such families more frequently exhibit alcoholism and/or psychopathy. One recent study attempted to factor out the relative importance of these

[7]Quite clearly this cannot apply to all alcoholic women, especially in this day of increasing sexual "emancipation." Many alcoholic women are quite self-confident and capable and often exhibit strong aggressive and ambitious drives, frequently occupying career roles that were traditionally the province of men. This complex psychosocial complexion among alcoholic women reflects a *potpourri* of "hyperfeminine" and acquiescent behavior together with an equal imperative toward individualism and "deviance" from feminine norms. [This is not to be construed in any way as a critical remark—deviance is an observable variation from a statistical norm, not a psychological or social criticism.]

psychiatric categories, along with gender and patterns of alcohol abuse (Gorenstein 1980). Because psychopathy is very rare among females and "hysteria" (histrionic personality) is thought by many investigators to be the female equivalent of male sociopathy (see Light 1986b), this diagnosis was also included in the study. Drinking patterns were categorized on the basis of (1) frequency of consumption per week, (2) amount of alcohol consumed per drinking episode, and (3) alcohol abuse, involving adverse consequences for the drinker—e.g., arrest, sickness and/or medical problems, loss of work or school time, social and interpersonal problems, etc., arising from alcohol abuse.

The results of Gorenstein's study support the traditional view that males drink significantly more alcohol than do females, despite claims to the contrary based upon the contention that the increasing "emancipation" of women is narrowing the differences between male and female drinking patterns. When the data for both sexes are combined, the general conclusion that depression and psychopathy are positively associated with abusive drinking is sustained. In addition, elevated depression and psychopathy scores are positively correlated with frequency of alcohol consumption (but not amount consumed per episode) in non-alcoholic individuals. However, when the data for males and females are considered separately, some rather striking differences emerge. Among males, both depression and psychopathy are positively associated with alcohol consumption. But depression is specifically associated with frequency of alcohol consumption (number of drinking days per week), suggesting that sustained drinking may function partly to "medicate" a chronic depressive affect. Psychopathy, on the other hand, appears to correlate with both frequency of drinking and quantity of alcohol consumed on each drinking occasion. This last pattern may reflect a greater tendency for impulsiveness and hedonism among psychopathically inclined males. Among females, neither depression nor psychopathy correlate with simple consumption indices, although both are significantly associated with alcohol abuse as indicated by negative consequences of drinking. However, hysteria is significantly correlated with sporadic "binge" drinking, suggesting at least a partial similarity between this psychiatric variant and psychopathy in males.

Isolation is a common feature among both male and female alcoholics, but it appears to be more severe for women who drink alone far more often and suffer more social isolation (Gomberg 1979). They also appear to exhibit significantly greater improvement in interpersonal relationships following recovery than do men. This suggests that such alcoholism-associated isolation in women may reflect an externally imposed exclusion because of the greater social rejection of female inebriates relative to males. Although alcoholic women do show evidence of somewhat greater psychopathology as discussed above, in several ways they exhibit a greater independence and sense of personal responsibility than do their male counterparts. Women alcoholics show much more concern about the welfare of their children than do males and they are much more likely to present themselves alone at alcoholism treatment facilities than are men (Gomberg 1979). That is, men are far more often accompanied by their wives than are women by their husbands.

Kinsey (1966) in a landmark social psychological study of alcoholism in women reported a bimodal age distribution for female inebriation patterns with peaks in the early thirties and early forties. Most of these women were concentrated in the 45 to 49 or in the 30 to 34 age brackets. His sample typically began drinking when approximately 18 years old and the mean age when first experiencing intoxication was about 22 years. However, at least 60 percent of these women became "tight" within one year after their first drink. And three out of four of his subjects who took their first drink as a child (defined as under 14) exhibited alcoholic symptoms prior to age 21. For those women who first began to drink before age 22, the mean age of onset of alcoholic symptoms was 31 to 32—about 9.8 years after the mean age when first intoxicated. For those who had their first drink after age 22, the mean difference between the age when first drunk and the onset of alcoholic symptoms was 6.7 years, thus showing the "telescoping effect" for alcoholic progression among women who begin to drink in later adulthood. Those women who begin drinking in their middle or late twenties progress more rapidly into alcoholic drinking, thus supporting the general impression about female alcoholism. He found three basic drinking patterns among women: (1) early initiation of drinking, usually late adolescence, with heavy drinking almost from the start and alcoholic symptoms appearing prior to age 20; (2) early onset of drinking followed by prolonged heavy social drinking and first alcoholic symptoms appearing in the early thirties; and (3) later onset of first drinking, usually in the late twenties followed by rapid progression into alcoholic drinking—half of these women experienced alcoholic symptoms within *two years* after their first experience with alcohol!

Cahalan *et al.* (1969, *in* Gomberg 1979) revealed that both men and women show a peak of heavy drinking between ages 45 through 49; in addition, women show an earlier peak of heavy drinking from ages 21 through 24. Other studies have shown that typical ranges for the onset of problem drinking in women is from 30 to 39, as compared to men in which the onset of problem drinking peaks from about age 27 to 32 (cited in Corrigan 1980). As Corrigan noted, telescoped alcoholic progression as reported for women has two components: (1) the shift from abstinence or moderate drinking to alcoholic drinking, and (2) the duration of alcoholic drinking until the patient is first seen at a hospital or clinic. Corrigan's study suggests that although women do first begin to drink later in life than men, the period of time between the first drink and the onset of problem drinking is not significantly different between the sexes—this sample reflected a mean age for the first drink of 21 and a mean onset of problem drinking at age 33. She was unable to confirm or deny that either component of telescoped progression existed in her sample, primarily because of uncertainty about statistics for the general population (see for example, the above conflicting data).

To further complicate matters, very young persons of both sexes are abusing alcohol and other drugs in escalating proportions, and the evidence is that there is little difference in drinking behavior between the sexes at these younger age levels (Corrigan 1980). As of the mid-1970's, 93 percent of boys and 87 percent of all girls had begun to drink by their last year in high school. For both sexes, adolescent crises are profound for many social and cultural reasons, and the rapid onset of florid alcoholism and other drug problems is increasing at an alarming rate. In the case of girls, when alcohol is the first drug of preference, telescoping appears to be maximal (Gomberg 1979). There is no question that more and more youngsters barely beyond adolescence are appearing for help at Alcoholics Anonymous with "drunkalogues" that rival those of their middle-aged counterparts with years more alcoholic drinking under their belts. It is my general impression that the majority of these young people are women, which may perhaps reflect the often reported tendency for females to seek help earlier than do men.[8] The common pattern of polydrug abuse among young people today both contributes to and results from the severe psychopathology seen in this group.

Corrigan's recent study (1980) regarding female alcoholism reported a number of interesting findings, including the following:

(1) The mean age at which the women in this study began drinking

[8]It has been the increasing trend in recent years for younger people of both sexes to join AA after brief but often virulent alcoholic careers. The demographic and epidemiological parameters of alcoholism are clearly undergoing rapid change.

was 21. Problem drinking was apparent by age 33 and it began earliest for those women who never married (age 30) and latest for widows (age 40). This study confirms earlier reports that women on the whole begin drinking at an earlier age than men, but in this case there was no apparent telescoping among the women relative to men.

(2) Women are more likely to be daily drinkers (two-thirds) than binge drinkers (28%); they generally consume slightly more than 11 drinks per day. Those who consume less than five drinks per day tend to have drunk more in the past, although rarely more than five to seven drinks per day.

(3) Urban women and particularly urban nonprofessional women are the heaviest drinkers. Professional women drink more often in bars and restaurants than do nonprofessional women, as do white women more often than black women, Catholic women more than Protestant women, and women of higher than lower socioeconomic status.

(4) Women tend to drink hard liquor rather than wine or beer, and 84 percent of them drink most often at home.

(5) Contrary to earlier reports, only 51 percent of alcoholic women relate the onset of alcoholic drinking to one or more specific life events. Once problem drinking has begun, two major reasons are associated with its persistence: (a) relief from feelings of anxiety, depression, unhappiness or loneliness, and (b) the pleasant and euphoric escape provided by alcohol.

(6) Both employed and unemployed married women and unmarried employed women are more likely to drink alone. Drinking alone is also associated with higher socioeconomic status. It is suggested that those women with strong attachments to others through marriage or employment are more inclined to maintain secrecy about their drinking.

(7) More than one-half of the women drink with others in their neighborhood, but they drink less than usual when drinking with neighbors, co-workers and members of their own family. They tend not to drink with people from their church but drink their usual amount only with close friends.

(8) The great majority of alcoholic women (82%!) have abused other drugs at some time during their lives, and nearly one-half have done so while drinking alcohol. Of those women who have used other drugs *while* drinking, 42 percent have used tranquilizers and sedatives, 24 percent have used sleeping medications, and 15 percent have used stimulants. White women, those under age 30, and very heavy drinkers are the most likely to use other drugs and to use other drugs while drinking. White

women are more likely to use other depressants and/or stimulants than are black women, and blacks are less likely than whites to use any other drug than alcohol. Women in general are less likely than men to use opiates, cocaine, or hallucinogens and there are no racial differences in this study for the use of these drugs.

(9) Those young women under 30 and those who consume 15 or more drinks per day are the most likely to use other drugs *together* with alcohol and who run the greatest risk of a lethal overdose combination of drugs.

(10) Most women tend to seek treatment within a short period after the onset of alcoholic drinking—typically within five or six years, or by an average age of 38.

Since this study involved female subjects who had already entered into treatment for their alcoholism in hospitals, clinics, and Alcoholics Anonymous, it is difficult to extrapolate the relevance of the above findings to the general population of alcoholic women. Both men and women who are recovering or who have recovered from alcoholism represent the mere tip of the famous iceberg of the problem at large. Futhermore, it takes a very special kind of courage and personal strength to be able to acknowledge an alcohol problem and be willing to do something about it. Alcoholic men and women in recovery are almost certainly unlike their still practicing peers in a number of ways—for every individual that recovers, between 20 and 30 others will ultimately die of their alcoholism and its complications. On the other hand, it is true that an ever increasing proportion of alcoholic men and women *are* entering into recovery, due in no small part to the massive educational campaigns in recent years that has made recovery resources much more available to the general population. These findings are intriguing, but like the earlier studies, their significance should be viewed with at least somc caution.

A number of studies have shown that women attain higher blood alcohol levels (BAL's) than do men at equivalent doses of alcohol and they become more intoxicated than men at the same dose of alcohol per unit body weight (Gomberg 1979). This is partly accounted for by the smaller volume of distribution of ethanol for females relative to males resulting from the greater amount of body fat generally found in women (see Light 1985). Although this body fat does sequester out a greater proportion of the ethanol from the blood than in males after a sufficient period of time and number of passages of the blood through the body has occurred, the elevated concentration of blood alcohol on the rising part of the BAL curve inevitably leads to enhanced disruption of neural membrane architecture and increased intoxication. Because of the steeper rise and higher BAL peak and the subsequently greater sequestering of alcohol in the fat stores, women tend to become drunker on similar doses of alcohol, but they also sober up more quickly.[9] Women also normally have a smaller concentration of red blood cells than men, the mean *hematocrit* or packed cell volumes being 42 percent of the blood volume and 47 percent, respectively (Bowman and Rand 1980).[10] The whole blood to plasma ratio of ethanol is 1:1.18 for a normal hematocrit value; for an individual with a lower hematocrit the same blood concentration of ethanol would amount to a higher plasma concentration of the drug *(loc. cit.)* It is the *plasma* concentration of a drug that is the true measure of pharmacological efficacy, and it is the criterion usually employed with drugs other than alcohol.

Among individual males BAL peaks tend to be fairly constant from test to test for a given dose of ethanol. On the other hand the female BAL response varies considerably more than in males from test to test in response to changes during the estrous cycle (Gomberg 1979; Ghodse and Tregenza 1980). BAL profiles increase during the premenstrual and ovulation phases and decrease during other phases of the cycle. This does support reports linking increased alcohol intake by women during periods of premenstrual tension. Premenstrual tension in itself is associated with emotional conflict, and the various menstrual symptoms reported by alcoholic women such as dysmennorrhea, fainting, blushing, etc., may result from a chronic emotional state of tension. Somatoform complaints of this type are particularly common in histrionic and depressed women—both diagnostic categories which are commonly seen among alcoholic women. Premenstrual discomfort and tension may thus result from the underlying emotional conflicts accompanying alcoholism, and at the same time feed back into those same conflicts and reinforce the symptomatic drinking.

Women taking oral contraceptives metabolize alcohol more slowly, but also more regularly and predictably than those not taking such medica-

[9]There is some evidence that alcohol metabolism is in general faster in women than in men (Ghodse and Tregenza 1980).

[10]Plasma is the liquid portion of the blood in which the formed elements or corpuscles are suspended. The hematocrit is determined by centrifuging a sample of the blood in a tube so that the erythrocytes are sedimented out to form a packed cell volume at the bottom. The percentage of the packed cell volume to the total volume of blood in the tube is the hematocrit.

tions. Chronic alcohol abuse and ensuing liver damage is consistently associated with significantly lowered testosterone and elevated estrogen levels in alcoholic males (Lieber 1983). The implications of this are intriguing, especially in view of the fact that premenopausal women under age 45 are more likely to develop liver cirrhosis than are either male or postmenopausal female alcoholics (Ghodse and Tregenza 1980).

Several gynecological and obstetrical problems appear to be associated with alcoholism in women: infertility, miscarriages, hysterectomies, difficult birth, and problems in conception and carrying to term being especially common.[11]

Seventy-eight percent of alcoholic women report such problems as compared to 35 percent of controls (Gomberg 1980). The same comments with regard to whether the symptoms precipitate or result from the alcohol abuse apply here, and a complex pattern of mutually reinforcing symptoms, consequent behaviors, and subsequent symptomatic exacerbation appears to prevail. Despite the popular association of female alcoholism with sexual promiscuity, the characteristic sexual problem seen among alcoholic women is frigidity (Gomberg 1980).

[11]The reader is also referred to the chapter on fetal alcohol syndrome.

GENETIC FACTORS IN ALCOHOLISM AND ASSOCIATED DISORDERS

THE EVIDENCE is rapidly becoming increasingly clear and compelling that most of the major psychiatric disorders, including alcoholism, are genetically inherited. This is certainly true for the mood disturbances (mania, hypomania and depression), alcoholism (which is closely related to affective disorder), schizophrenias, and even sociopathy (antisocial personality disorder). And there is growing suspicion that this may be true of many neurotic disorders, as well. Furthermore, several studies have revealed that identical twins reared apart from one another show startling similarities in their personalities, lifestyles and even the names of their spouses, children and pets (see Light 1985). In this chapter we will review the evidence supporting these concentrations and provide the genetically unsophisticated reader with enough background in the subject to enable him to comprehend the significance of the emerging research reports.

At the risk of being tedious (see also Light 1985, 1986b) I wish to emphasize once again as strongly as I can that the continuing and often acrimonious conflict between the "nature and nurture" schools of human personality and development is a red herring. Just because a major portion of who one is and how he or she behaves is under strong genetic control by no means implies that one's cultural, social and family environment plays no role. Alcoholics, for example, typically come from broken homes and disrupted family backgrounds, and this can hardly have little or no effect upon the developing child. Active alcoholism in the family of a developing child will certainly have an adverse impact upon him, such that he inevitably develops pathological and inappropriate coping behaviors in response to a grossly destructive environment. Such children all too frequently grow up to become alcoholics themselves or co-alcoholics exhibiting a lifelong, pathological involvement with other alcoholics, sociopaths, or other seriously impaired individuals. These unfortunates know no other way to exist. Because they have always lived under such circumference they cannot help but operate from the premise that one can *only* survive in similar circumstances.

But psychiatrically impaired adults also tend to be genetically and biologically vulnerable to psychological damage due to these adverse circumstances. In fact, they often develop psychiatric problems even in the absence of a pathological family or social setting. All of us experience a great many stresses and personal tragedies in the course of growing up, although some are clearly buffeted by much more extreme trauma than others. Psychologically healthy individuals are much more able to let these traumatic events and circumstances roll off their backs than those susceptible to psychological decompensation. Even traumatic stress responses to devastating life events (war, natural disaster, concentration camp experiences, etc.) appear to be more extreme in psychiatrically vulnerable individuals than in healthy individuals. Vulnerable persons are much more likely to react to the vicissitudes of living (loss of job, career setback, divorce, death of a spouse or child, etc.) with severe and prolonged depression and functional paralysis than are normal individuals. The latter tend to go through a period of normal mourning after which they are again able to function well and to handle their responsibilities appropriately.

In order to properly understand the many facets of psychiatric disturbances in general and of alcoholism in particular, one must fully comprehend the many biological, psychosocial and spiritual factors that underlie them. It is truly regrettable that so many academics and professional clinicians appear to be so intractably mired in the rigid insistence that a particular phenomenon must be *either* biologically *or* psychosocially determined. Academics and intellectuals have an almost phobic aversion for ambiguity and what appears to be logical inconsistency. Their world views are largely confined to the narrow constraints of a particular theory or model to which they are attached. Psychologists and sociologists tend to reject strongly any suggestion that biology or heredity plays a significant role, primarily because these factors lie outside their own disciplines. This narrow-minded view reaches its extreme expression in Stanton Peele's insistence that the chemical addictions have absolutely no biological foundation whatsoever and that even physical addiction is in no way related to the biological activity of a drug (Peele 1981).

Such intellectual tunnel-vision by the proponents of alternative models of the etiologies of psychiatric disorders not only leads to needless, disruptive and irrelevant arguments in the professional and popular media. Deplorably, it also results in the wholesale rejection by the proponents of one school of very meritorious and useful ideas coming from opposing camps. A case in point can be seen in Peele's insistence that biology plays no role in the development of addiction. This assertion is patently absurd, yet much of the rest of his theory of addiction is very apt and to the point. His description of addiction as a manifestation of inappropriately channeled love reflecting the individual's sense of powerlessness over his life and circumstances is a powerful insight.

Addictions are manifestations of extremely complex, multifactorial processes.[12] Any comprehensive model of the addictions must include all of the factors and dynamics that are known to be causally related to or which otherwise impinge upon and affect them.

And finally, it must be said that strict adherence to logical consistency cannot provide an adequate description of the Universe. Both the theory of relativity and quantum mechanics are accepted as if not actually true,[13] then as the best and most useful model of how things are by nearly all competent scientists in the world today. Nature is revealed as fundamentally "dualistic." Our logic and our self-consistent science have led us into the strange situation in which mutually contradictory states which cannot simultaneously exist within a single system have been conclusively demonstrated to do just that! The fundamental, "real" nature of matter appears to be far more bizarre and improbable than any science-fantasy writer could have dreamed up on his or her own. Matter

[12] I make no inferences regarding the nature and etiological processes underlying the non-substance addictions such as compulsive gambling, videoarcade mania and the eating disorders. I do not pretend to understand these disorders and I have no view as to whether they are or are not related to substance abuse. Superficial resemblance and symptomatology does not necessarily mean that the underlying causes are the same. Nevertheless, even the non-substance addictions exhibit the major distinguishing feature which characterizes addictions in general: the addictive behavior *does something for the addict* that it does not do for non-addicts. It produces a temporary state of euphoria and/or relief from stress and dysphoria—and this effect may well be mediated by biological factors.

[13] In science and philosophy nothing can ever be unequivocally demonstrated as being "true" or as an accurate model of objective reality. In the first place, a scientific model can only be said to be a "useful" model of reality if it is self-consistent and compatible with all other accepted scientific "fact" and theory, and after it has successfully withstood the tests of all experiments performed to ascertain its validity. Secondly, relativity theory and quantum physics, both of which have always been demonstrated to be "true" by all available scientific evidence, inevitably lead to logical inconsistency and paradox. Matter, for example, cannot simultaneously have both a particle-nature and a wave-nature, yet this is clearly the case. The "true" answer one always obtains in any quantum mechanical experiment is inevitably determined by the question one happens to ask. "Is the photon a particle?" or "Is it a wave?" will always result in a "yes" answer to whichever question is put to Nature. Similarly, "Is alcoholism a biological disorder?" or "Is it a psychosocial one?" will always be answered in the affirmative regardless of which question is being asked.

can be equally well described in terms of its particle-nature on the one hand, and on the basis of its wavelike properties on the other. Similarly, alcoholics and at least several other so-called "behavioral" disorders are now known to arise from a complex interaction between genetic and environmental factors. To regard these disorders from only one perspective will provide only an incomplete and fragmented picture of what are in reality heterogeneous entities with multiple etiologies. This caveat aside, and by now I trust thoroughly understood, let us begin our discussion of the genetic factors involved in the etiology of alcoholism and certain associated neuropsychiatric states. The psychodynamic factors have been given full treatment elsewhere (Light 1986b).

Overview of Biochemical Genetics

The chemical substance which carries the hereditary information which determines the sum total of a cell's biochemical functions and structural architecture is *deoxyribonucleic acid* or *DNA*. DNA is made up of a ladder-like double helix of nitrogen-bearing *bases,* each attached to a *pentose* (5-carbon) sugar, *deoxyribose,* which is in turn attached to two phosphate groups (Figure 1). Each base-deoxyribose-phosphate unit is known as a *nucleotide.* The nucleotides are arranged sequentially along a pair of backbones consisting of deoxyribose units connected to the phosphate groups by phosphodiester bonds. The nitrogenous bases attached to the deoxyribose units protrude from and connect the two parallel sugar-phosphate strands in a ladder-like series of "rungs" consisting of paired bases joined by *hydrogen bonds.*[14] The bases consist of single or double ring structures known as *pyrimidines* and *purines,* respectively. Adenosine is a *nucleoside* (a base plus deoxyribose) containing *adenine* (Figure 1), one of the two purines found in DNA (the other being *guanine*). The two *pyrimidines* are *thymine* and *cytosine* (Figure 1). Because of the difference in size between the purines and pyrimidines, in order for the two stands of helical backbone to remain parallel, each purine must be hydrogen-bonded to one of the pyrimindines, and vice versa. Specifically, adenine can only hydrogen-bond to thymine, and cytosine only to guanine.

[14]Hydrogen bonds are formed when hydrogen is covalently bonded to a strongly electronegative atom such as oxygen or nitrogen. The electronegative atom strongly attracts the electrons away from the hydrogen atom so that the latter is left as a more or less naked proton. This positively-charged proton then forms a weak electrostatic attraction with a negatively charged region on another molecule. This weak electrostatic attraction constitutes a hydrogen bond.

The nucleotides form extremely long, paired, polynucleotide sequences forming the double-stranded helical DNA chain joined to one another by the base-base rungs held together by hydrogen bonds (Figure 1). DNA replicates itself by "unzipping" the hydrogen bonds between the base-base pairs so that the two DNA polynucleotide strands separate and unwind (Figure 2). The bases of each separated strand are thus exposed directly to the surrounding medium. These unpaired bases attract their respective complementary nucleotides from the surrounding nucleoplasm[15] so that an exact complementary strand forms on each exposed strand from the original paired strands of the DNA double-helix. The result is two new double strands of DNA exactly like the original, with one of the original strands being present in each daughter strand. During normal cell division one of the daughter strands will go to each daughter cell. This insures that each cell receives an exact copy of the original DNA strand. The unzipping process and the formation of complementary nucleotide strands are catalyzed by enzymes known as *DNA polymerases.*

DNA molecules also are the templates from which complementary nucleotide strands known as *ribonucleic acid* or *mRNA* are synthesized. RNA (Figure 2) is very much like DNA except that the pentose sugar, *ribose,* (Figure 1B) contains one more oxygen atom than does deoxyribose (Figure 1A). Furthermore, the pyrimidine base thymine in DNA is replaced by *uracil* in RNA. RNA is synthesized along a naked strand of DNA in exactly the same manner as complementary DNA, except that the process is initiated by *RNA polymerase* (Figure 2). DNA self-replicates during the process of cell division to provide each daughter cell with precisely the same DNA content and arrangement as existed in the parent cell. RNA synthesis is initiated for the purpose of translating the genetic information contained in the DNA into the production of specific proteins.

The basic unit of heredity is the *gene,* a long sequence of DNA[16] containing about a hundred to more than a thousand nucleotides. Each gene codes for a specific protein and each is characterized by a specific sequence of nucleotides. It is the exact sequence of nucleotides that provides the code for protein synthesis. Each protein consists of a highly specific sequence of amino acids (see Light 1985) linked together by

[15] In eukaryotic cells the DNA is contained within a membrane-enclosed nucleus and the nuclear protoplasmic medium is called the *nucleoplasm.*

[16] Some viruses contain RNA instead of DNA in their genomes.

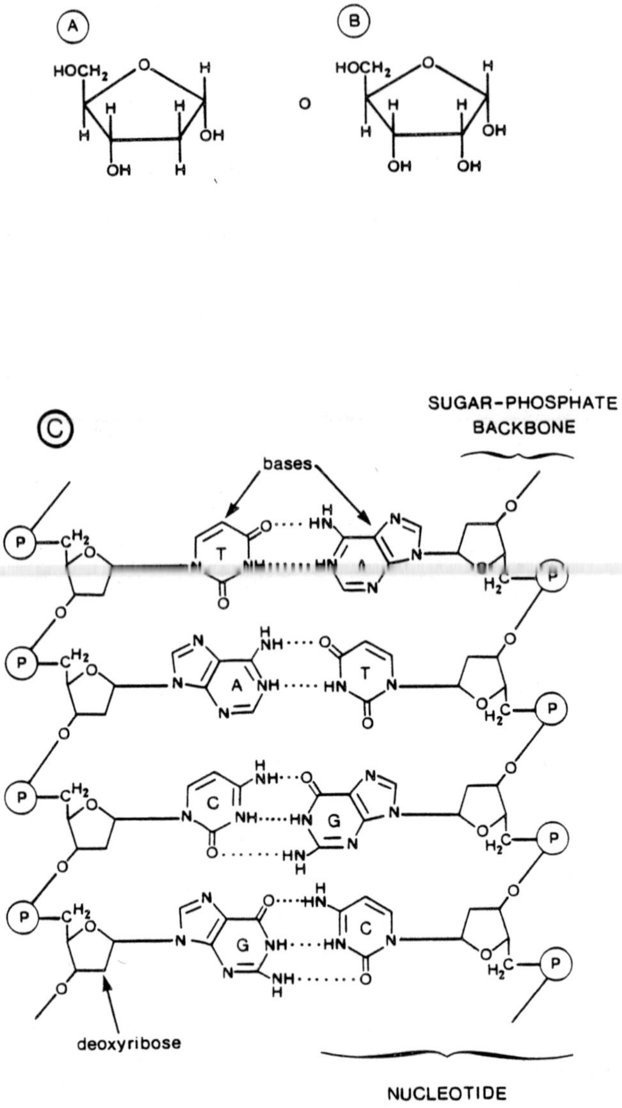

Figure 1. The Strucutre of DNA. A. The pentose (5-carbon) sugar deoxyribose, which is found in deoxyribonucleic acid (DNA). **B.** The pentose sugar ribose, which contains one more oxygen atom than does deoxyribose, and which occurs in ribonucleic acid (RNA). **C.** DNA is made up of two deoxyribose-phosphate backbones wound around each other in a double helix (see Figure 2), with an inward protruding nitrogenous base attached to each sugar molecule. Each base-sugar-phosphate unit constitutes a nucleotide. Each base attached to one of the phosphate-sugar backbones is hydrogen-bonded to its counterpart from the opposite backbone, forming a ladderlike series of "rungs." The bases consist of single- or double-ring structures known respectively as pyrimidines and purines. The two pyrimidines found in DNA are thymine (T) and cytosine (C), and the two purines are adenine (A) and guanine (G). [In RNA, thymine is replaced by another pyrimidine base, uracil.] Because of the size differences between the two classes of bases, each pyrimidine is hydrogen-bonded to a purine in order for the backbones to remain parallel. Specifically, adenine is always associated with thymine, and cytosine only with guanine.

peptide bonds. Proteins are accordingly also called *polypeptides,* and the exact arrangement of the amino acids gives the protein its specific functional or structural activity. The synthesis of proteins from DNA templates is mediated by several different types of RNA, each of which has a specific structure and function.

In eukaryotic cells *messenger RNA (mRNA)* carries the genetic information from the DNA template out of the nucleus and into the cytoplasm to the ribosomes where protein synthesis occurs (Figure 2). The complementary RNA that forms along naked strands of DNA in reponse to RNA polymerase in such cells is mRNA. This mRNA is a negative cast, as it were, of the positive mold provided by DNA. This complementary transcript (the process of mRNA synthesis along a DNA template is called *transcription*) moves out of the nucleus and attaches to ribosomes in the cytoplasm, the latter consisting of about two thirds *ribosomal RNA (rRNA)* and one third protein. The ribosomes are the factories where polypeptides or proteins are fashioned out of amino acids. The mRNA molecules function as messengers which convey the genetic information contained in the DNA to the protein synthesizing machinery, the ribosomes, where specific polypeptides are formed, these being the end product of the genes. The process by which the coded information on mRNA is converted into specific amino acid sequences is termed *translation.*

In prokaryotic organisms mRNA begins to function in translation immediately after being synthesized from the DNA template. In mammals, however, including humans, the mRNA that ultimately enters the cytoplasm and activates the ribosomes is not that synthesized directly from DNA. The immediate products of gene transcription in mammals represent a distinct type of RNA which are very large and heterogeneous. These molecules are known as *heterogenous nuclear RNA (hnRNA)* or simply as *nuclear RNA (nRNA).* Most of the hnRNA synthesized in the mammalian nucleus is degraded or undergoes a series of additions, deletions, cleavages and other modifications. Only a small portion of transcribed hnRNA actually becomes incorporated into mRNA in the cytoplasm and participates in the translation of the genetic code into proteins.

The actual translation of the gentic code into protein involves yet another kind of RNA known as *transfer* or *soluble RNA (tRNA),* the smallest variety consisting of only 70 to 80 nucleotides. Transfer RNA picks up individual amino acids drifting around in the cytoplasm, each tRNA selecting for a specific amino acid. A tRNA molecule is folded back

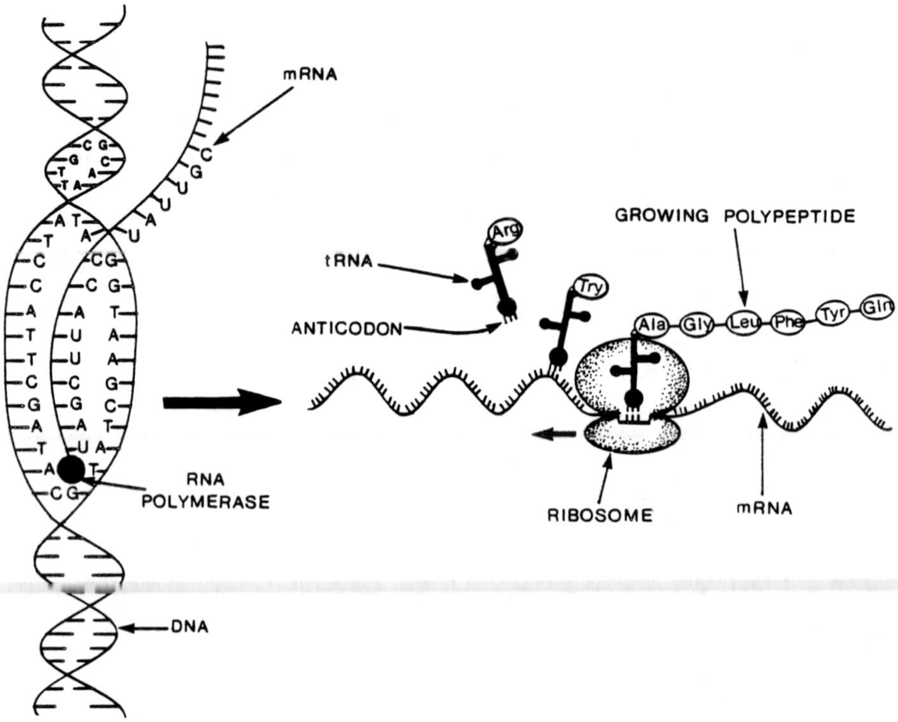

Figure 2. Protein Synthesis: Transcription and Translation. In transcription, messenger RNA (mRNA) is synthesized from one of DNA strands. This process begins when the enzyme RNA polymerase acts upon the promoter region (see Figure 11) of a specific sequence of nucleotides, causing the double-stranded DNA to unwind. The DNA directs the synthesis of mRNA by the process of complementary base-pairing (see text). In eukaryotic cells (those of all higher plants and animals), mRNA synthesis occurs inside the nucleus of the cell. The mRNA then leaves the nucleus and enters the cytoplasm where it attaches to the ribosomes, where protein synthesis (translation) actually takes place. The mRNA serves as the template for polypeptide synthesis. Amino acids in the cytoplasm combine with specific transfer RNA (tRNA) molecules, which bear a three-nucleotide sequence at one pole known as the anticodon. This anticodon is exactly complementary to a three-nucleotide codon on the mRNA, and as the mRNA "runs" through the ribosomes, one codon after another is sequentially presented to the corresponding tRNA molecules with their attached amino acids. Each amino acid is added to the prowing peptide chain in the exact order prescribed by the mRNA template, and the newly unencumbered tRNA molecule is released back into the cytoplasm where it can pick up another specific amino acid. The small arrow to the left of the ribosome in the above diagram represents the direction of movement of the ribosome relative to the mRNA chain. Although this figure shows only one amino acid-bearing tRNA attached to the ribosome, in fact there are two sites — the *p*- or peptide tRNA site and the *a*- or amino acid-binding site; both sites are occupied during translation.

upon itself in complex ways (Figure 2) and each bears a *3' A•C•C terminus* which attaches to an amino acid via an ester bond. The attachment of the amino acid requires a specific *aminoacyl-tRNA synthetase,* one for each of the 20 different amino acids. These enzymes recognize their specific tRNA molecule by means of the charge distributions on the latter. Each tRNA also bears a three-nucleotide sequence at one pole called the *anticodon* which is complementary to a similar sequence on mRNA known as the *codon.*

The ribosomes have three binding sites: two of these sites are for tRNA and one for mRNA. As the mRNA runs zipperlike along the ribosome each codon triplet codes for its complementary anticodon as it appears at the triple binding site. Thus, two specific tRNA molecules with their respective attached amino acids are brought into close proximity which allows for a peptide bond to form between the two amino acids, which thus add to the growing polypeptide chain. The sequence of amino acids in a protein are thus determined by the sequence of nucleotide bases fed through a ribosome. In this complex manner the genetic code is transcribed from DNA to mRNA, and the mRNA *translates* the code into protein synthesis by bringing specific tRNA molecules with their attached amino acids into close proximity so that peptide bonds can form.

Each gene typically codes for one specific protein (there are exceptions to this, see below). Because all biochemical reactions are catalyzed by enzymes, which are proteins, and because proteins form a major part of cell structure, the production of specific proteins at the right time and in the right place accounts for the entire diversity of all living things that have ever existed on this planet. If you change one nucleotide in a gene sequence, you will change the fundamental nature of the protein that is coded for by that gene. In fact, you will have induced a *mutation* in that gene which will result in a different end product.

Changes in the nucleotide sequence of DNA can occur in a variety of ways. Cytosine and adenine spontaneously deaminate (lose their amino groups) to form uracil and hypoxanthine, respectively. Because neither of these bases is normally found in DNA, special enzymes known as *endonucleases* are usually able to identify this defect and excise it. A *repair DNA polymerase* and a *ligase* acting in concert then return the DNA to its original state. A number of mutations occur in response to damaging chemicals or ultraviolet or other high-energy radiation. Radiation in particular can cause adjacent thymine bases in a DNA sequence to undergo a dimerization process in which the carbon double bonds within the ring system of each thymine molecule are broken to form bonds directly between the two bases. The ensuing dimer often results in a gap in the RNA transcription that forms from the DNA template, resulting in a change in the polypeptide sequence it orchestrates. The same kind of changes can occur in mRNA sequences after they form. If the repair mechanisms for restoring the nucleotide strands to their original state are defective or fail to operate, the mutation will be translated into the resulting protein which will then result in a change in the protein's biochemical activity.

The genes lie along vast strands of DNA. In the case of primitive prokaryotes the genes and the proteins for which they code are *colinear.* That is, the sequence of amino acids in a protein lie in exactly the same unbroken order as the sequence of codons (nucleotide triplets) in the gene which codes for it. In higher eukaryotic organisms the genes occur as a series of DNA sequences containing the genetic information separated by intervening groups of nonsense nucleotides called *intervening sequences.* Those separated fragments of polypeptide-coding DNA are termed *encoding sequences.*[17] Since the gene is the complete DNA sequence which codes for a specific polypeptide, the genes in higher organisms consist of the sum total of encoding sequences together with the intervening sequences necessary to produce a complete protein. Each protein therefore is made up of several shorter segments, each synthesized from different encoding sequences on the gene.

The entire DNA sequence, including the nonsense sections, is copied by the hnRNA that forms during transcription. This hnRNA is then "edited" by several different enzymes that variously cut out and delete the nonsense fragments, and splice the several encoding sequences together to produce a functional mRNA that leaves the nucleus, enters the cytoplasm and attaches to the ribosomes to initiate translation.

Overview of Classical Genetics

The DNA of higher organisms is contained within dark-staining, rod-like structures called *chromosomes* (Figure 3). The chromosomes consist of both nucleic acid and protein and are contained within the nucleus of the cell. All of the genes which code for proteins in an organism are contained within these chromosomes, and each gene occupies a specific site

[17]Most viral DNA also consists of encoding sequences interrupted by intervening sequences.

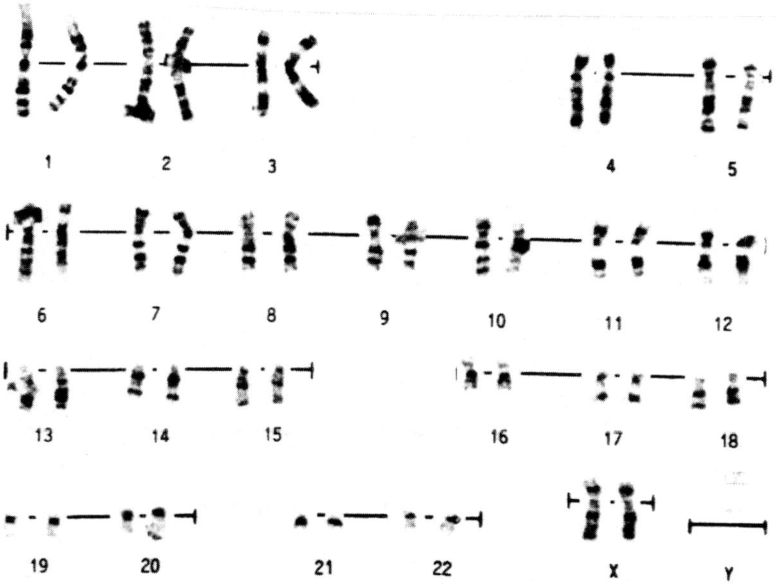

Figure 3. Human Karyotype. A normal female human karyotype with 22 autosomes and two X-chromosomes. The homologous pairs are numbered and each pair contains one chromosome from each parent. The above figure is the karyotype of the author's youngest daughter, courtesy of Dr. George Henry and David Peakman of the Cytogenetics Laboratory, Reproductive Genetics Center in Denver, Colorado.

within a specific chromosome. All higher organisms have a specific number of chromosomes, half of which are derived from one parent and half from the other parent. The total number of chromosomes in human cells is 46, of which half, or 23, come from each parent. The total number and appearance of the chromosomes in a specific organism is known as the organism's *karyotype.* The total number of genes contained within a human cell is estimated at between 10,000 and 2.5 million (Tsuang and Vandermey 1980).

In humans there are 22 *homologous pairs* of *autosomes* and a pair of *sex chromosomes,* with one member of each pair coming from each parent. Each member of a homologous pair of chromosomes contains precisely the same genes coding for the same proteins located at precisely the same location (*locus*) in each chromosome. Thus, the gene for eye color is found in exactly the same place in each homologous chromosome. Although the genes from each parent at the same locus on homologous chromosomes are the same (for eye color, for example), they may or may not code for the same color. The corresponding genes at a given locus in homologous chromosomes are called *alleles*; one allele of a gene pair may code for blue eyes, and the other for brown. Some genes may exist as several different alleles, all coding for different expressions (traits) of a given feature (eye color, hair color, presence or absence of specific enzyme activity, etc.), whereas others only exist as one allele. There are alleles which confer relative immunity to malaria, but which also produce sickle-cell trait, for example.

When identical alleles are present for each gene of a homologous pair (two alleles for blue eyes, for example) the individual is *homozygous* for that trait; if the alleles code for different expressions of the trait (one allele codes for blue, the other for brown), the individual is *heterozygous* for that trait. Very commonly one allele will overrule another in determining the feature that actually appears in the individual. For example, when a person is heterozygous for eye color, that is containing an allele for blue and an allele for brown, the eye color that appears in the fully formed individual will be brown. The brown allele overwhelms the blue allele. The brown allele is said to be *dominant* and the blue allele is *recessive.* Thus, when an individual is homozygous dominant (that is, it has two dominant alleles—brown + brown) or is heterozygous (has brown + blue), the eye color actually expressed will be brown. Blue eyes will appear only if the person is homozygous recessive (blue + blue). The entire complement of genes carried by an individual is termed that individual's *genotype;* the actual overt physical expression that appears in the individual is called his *phenotype.* Thus, an individual's genotype might be heterozygous (brown-blue) and his phenotype dominant brown. See also Appendix 1.

The two sex chromosomes determine the indivudal's gender. Two X-chromosomes will produce a female whereas an X- and a Y-chromosome will result in a male. Because females have only X-chromosomes, they can only donate an X-chromosome to their offspring (about which more below). Males, on the other hand, can donate either an X- or a Y-chromosome. It is therefore the male, all other things being equal,[18] that determines the sex of the offspring. Although the X- and Y-chromosomes are homologous, the Y-chromosome lacks most of the short arm which is present on the X-chromosome.[19] Therefore, the XY or

---

[18]Other factors, such as vaginal pH which may differentially affect X- and Y-carrying spermatozoa, may originate in the female, who may thus also help determine the sex of the offspring.

[19]Each chromosome has two arms joined usually at a central point called the *centromere* or *kinetochore;* however, in some chromosomes the kinetochore is located very near one end so that the short arm is almost indistinguishable. The kinetochore provides a point of attachment for the spindle fibers (see Appendix 1) which act to draw the members of homologous pairs apart during cell division.

male condition provides that all of the genes carried by the short arm of the X-chromosome have no Y-counterpart. Therefore only one allele is present for each of these genes. This is termed the *hemizygous* condition and those traits which are carried by the X- but not the Y-chromosome are known as *sex-linked traits*. Because of this hemizygosity, recessive alleles carried by the short arm of the X-chromosome are expressed by the phenotype because there is no countering allele on the Y-chromosome. Hemizygous males therefore tend to express sex-linked recessive traits. Females, which bear two X-chromosomes, will express the dominant phenotype when their genotype is heterozygous for the trait.

Red-green colorblindness and haemophilia are both sex-linked recessive traits in human beings. Thus, although females can be carriers of the trait, only males can express it in the phenotype. Because of the way in which the genes segregate out during germ cell maturation (see Appendix 1), if a woman who is heterozygous for a sex-linked recessive trait mates with a normal man, one-half of the sons produced by this pair would show the phenotype—that is, be color-blind or have haemophilia. And one-half of the daughters would carry the trait. None of the daughters could express the phenotype. This could happen only if the daughter also inherited the same recessive allele from the other parent, something that could happen only if the father overtly expressed the trait in his phenotype.

Sex-linked dominant inheritance can also occur. The presence of a dominant allele on the X-chromosome in male offspring or on either of the X-chromosomes in female offspring will result in overt phenotypic expression of the trait (*complete penetrance*). Because the father can only transmit a Y-chromosome to his sons (see Appendix 1 for a brief review of meiosis and gene segregation), none of his sons will carry or express the trait despite the fact that the father does, unless the mother donates an X-chromosome with the trait to the son. In either case, both parents of a son with the phenotype for the trait will also express the phenotype. Distinguishing between an X-linked dominant trait and autosomal dominant inheritance (see below) is very difficult. Sex-linked dominant inheritance may operate in families exhibiting bipolar disorder and "unipolar" depression also occurring in such families. It does not appear to operate in those families exhibiting only unipolar depression. Vitamin D-resistant rickets with hypophosphatemia is another example of X-linked dominant inheritance in humans.

Most genes are carried on the autosomes and single-gene inheritance (the phenotypic expression of a trait is carried by a single gene at a single locus on a specific chromosome) is therefore usually *autosomal-dominant* or *autosomal-recessive.* Individuals who are homozygous-dominant for an autosomal trait will produce only gametes bearing the dominant allele, and all of their offspring will therefore express the trait in their phenotype (see Appendix 1). If both parents are heterozygous for the trait, one out of four of their offspring will be homozygous-dominant, one will be homozygous-recessive, and two will be heterozygous. Therefore, three out of every four children will express the trait and one will not (see the Punnet square in Appendix 1). Clearly, homozygous parents can only pass the allele for which they are homozygous to their offspring.

Autosomal recessive traits can only be expressed in the phenotype when the individual is homozygous for the allele. Individuals who are heterozygous for a recessive trait are *carriers* of that trait. Half the gametes produced by a heterozygous parent will carry the recessive trait and half will have the dominant one. If these germ cells combine with those from a homozygous dominant parent, one half the offspring will be carriers but none will express the trait phenotypically. If a heterozygote mates with another heterozygote, one of four of the offspring will be homozygous dominant, one will be homozygous recessive, and two will be heterozygous (see Appendix 1 and the discussion of Punnet squares). Therefore, only one out of every four offspring of two heterozygous parents will express the trait phenotypically. The offspring of parents, one of which is homozygous dominant and the other homozygous recessive, will all be heterozygous and express the dominant allele phenotypically. Both autosomal dominant and autosomal recessive traits are inherited equally often by both sexes. It should be clear that autosomal recessive traits can be carried cryptically for several generations without being expressed in the phenotype, only to surface suddenly in a homozygous recessive descendant.

The simple dominant-recessive type of Mendelian[20] inheritance we have discussed thus far is more often the exception than the rule. Many genes exhibit *incomplete dominance* in heterozygotic offspring as seen, for example in certain types of cattle. Crosses between a homozygous-recessive (white animal) and a homozygous-dominant (red animal) may yield one homozygous-recessive, white calf, one homozygous-dominant, red calf, and two heterozygous intermediates or roan-colored calves.

[20]Gregor Mendel, an Augustinian monk in a part of Austria currently under Czechoslovakian control, published an obscure paper in 1866 about breeding experiments he had conducted on peas. His work, which was rediscovered at the turn of the century, revealed the statistical patterns of inheritance which bear his name and which is briefly discussed here and in Appendix 1.

Furthermore, some alleles may behave as dominant genes in one sex but as recessive ones in the other. Such genes are termed *sex-limited.* Male-pattern baldness is an example.

Many genes exist as more than just two alleles. Such genes are said to have *multiple alleles.* Each allele in such a multiple allele system represents a variation of the same gene. Therefore a given individual can possess only two of these alleles. The A-B-O system of human blood types is a multiple allele system.[21] There are three alleles which determine human blood types: I^A, I^B, and I^O. I^O is recessive and I^A and I^B are *codominant* relative to each other, that is the effects of both alleles are expressed equally in the heterozygous condition. The combinations I^A/I^A and I^A/I^O produce a Type A phenotype, I^B/I^B and I^B/I^O yield Type B, I^O/I^O results in a phenotype of Type O, and I^A/I^B gives rise to Type AB blood. Because I^O is recessive only four phenotypes are possible.

Most inherited traits are determined by more than just one gene. In many cases the phenotypic expression of one gene is influenced by one or more other genes known as *modifying genes.* The influence of one gene pair over another, nonallelomorphic[22] pair relative to the overall phenotypic expression or penetrance is called *epistasis.* The phenotypic manifestation of a gene may also be modified by other alleles at the same locus. This is illustrated by the differences in age of onset of a progressively deteriorating condition known as myotonic dystrophy. In this disorder, the penetrance of the abnormal dominant allele for myotonic dystrophy is significantly modified by the simultaneous presence of the normal allele from an unaffected parent. Some cases will thus present with an early onset and a severe, progressive deterioration, whereas others will develop later in life and run a more benign course.

A single gene may have multiple phenotypic expressions, a condition known as *pleiotropy.* Certain genetic mutations affecting red blood cells in man, for example, exhibit pleiotropy. Deficiencies in certain enzymes important in red blood cell glycolysis also affect other organ systems. Thus, a deficiency in red blood cell causes nonspherocytic hemolytic anemia (NSHA) and skeletal anomalies; in some patients the leucocytes as well as the erythrocytes are affected. Similarly, red blood cell phos-

[21] Human beings are classified into four basic blood groups: A, B, AB, and O. These groups differ from one another on the basis of specific antigens (see Light 1985) carried on the surface of red blood cells, which correspond to the presence or absence of specific enzymes. Some of these groups are incompatible with certain other groups, which may precipitate a serious and often fatal reaction in persons receiving the wrong type blood.

[22] Pairs of alleles at different loci relative to other gene pairs.

phofructokinase causes NSHA as well as severe myopathy and glycogen storage disorders and triosephosphate isomerase produces NSHA, neuromuscular anomalies, dementia and early death (data from Vogel and Motulsky 1979). Genes do not function primarily in isolation but work together to determine the overall phenotypic expression of the individual. Probably no gene affects only a single character, but may affect all other features. And probably no single phenotypic trait is produced by only one gene acting in isolation, but by many genes acting in concert against environmental parameters.

Multifactorial Inheritance

When many different genes combine to produce one phenotypic trait, inheritance is said to be *polygenic,* and when a given feature has many different phenotypic expressions, then the population is said to be *polymorphic* for that feature. Because genes never operate in a selective vacuum,[23] environmental variables play an important role in determining the eventual adult morphology (here interpreted to include biochemical activity as well as physical structure). The height to which an individual grows, for example, is determined by a great many genes all acting in concert, and selectively molded by the sum total of environmental parameters which the individual encounters as he grows up. The sum total of genetically determined biochemical activity operating at different times during the individual's growth (basic metabolism, hormonal activity, presence or lack of specific enzyme deficiency, etc.) operate against the background of the individual's environment. Nutritional factors, including availability in the diet of adequate protein, vitamins and minerals, pollution, degree of population pressure, altitude, and even such things as climate can all modify the genetic potential that an individual has, thus narrowing one's fundamental biological options to one degree or another.

Intelligence-quotient or IQ is another trait under such *multifactorial* influence. The individual's genetically determined, biological capacity to learn and integrate knowledge can be enhanced or curtailed by personality

[23]The sum total effect(s) of all environmental variables affecting an individual's well-being, including available food resources and shelter, competition for food, territory (or the economic equivalent) and sexual partner, exposure to disease or accident, and in the case of human societies at war or with high crime rates, predation, represent factors which select for or against the individual's likelihood of survival and reproduction. *Natural selection* is a fundamental mechanism thought to underlie the fitness and survival of individuals and species.

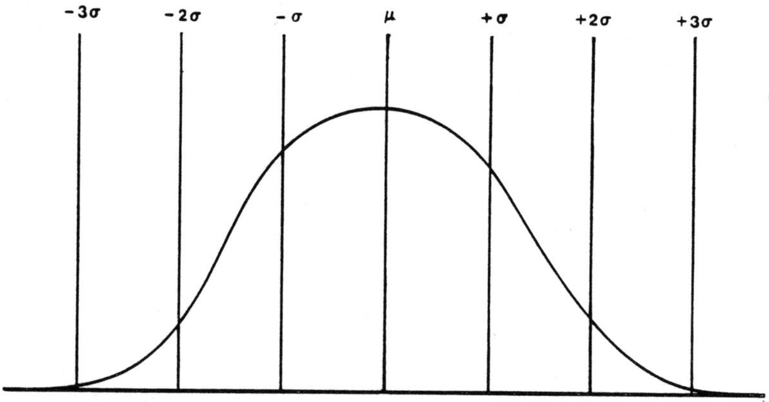

Figure 4. Normal Distribution of a Population of Measurements. In a normally distributed population of measurements (e.g., the heights of all 18-year-old males in the United States at any given time), most of the measurements will fall symmetrically about a central value known as the *mean*, μ—the arithmetic average of all measurements [$\mu = \Sigma X_i/N$, where N = the total number of measurements and X_i = the individual measurements in the population]. The symbols $\pm\sigma$, $\pm 2\sigma$, and $\pm 3\sigma$ represent 1, 2, and 3 standard deviations above and below the mean, respectively, as determined by the formula:

$$\sigma = \sqrt{\Sigma(X_i - \mu)^2/N}$$

In a normal population, 68.26 percent of all measurements will fall between $\pm\sigma$, 95.46 percent will fall between $\pm 2\sigma$, and 99.74 percent between $\pm 3\sigma$, respectively. In the above normal curve the horizontal axis represents the individual values of X_i and the vertical axis the frequency of each value of X_i. The vast majority of all measurements tend to cluster about the mean and the extreme deviations from the mean value are represented by only a few examples.

traits,[24] one's family, social and academic environment, peer pressure, and exposure to intellectual stimulation. All of these factors acting together are reflected in the tendency for most populations to exhibit a bell-shaped or *normal* frequency distribution (Figure 4) for any given trait. Such a curve reflects the fact that most statistical populations show a distinct aggregation of measurements about a central value. Most measurements thus lie within a fairly close value above or below the statistical mean (arithmetic average), with only a few lying at extreme values above and below the mean.

Many human diseases, including probably most neuropsychiatric ones, exhibit *multifactorial inheritance* with near relatives of patients with these disorders having an increased risk for developing the same disorder

[24]Devastating psychoses such as schizophrenia or childhood autism, for example, can completely overwhelm any innate biological intelligence one has so that they are unable to perform on any IQ test. Depression may also make an individual unable to actively learn or perform academically.

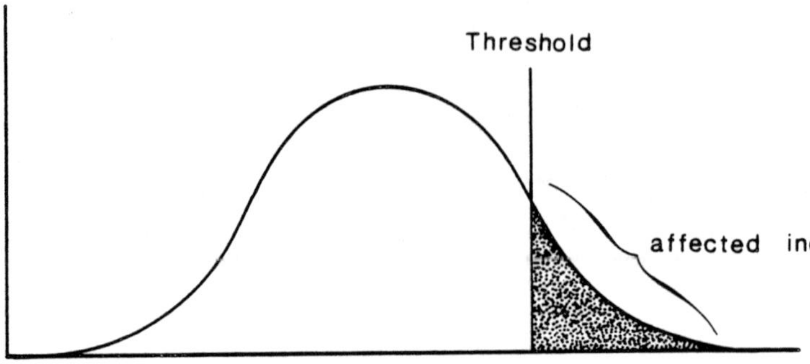

Figure 5. Multifactorial Inheritance With a Threshold Effect. The liability for developing a multifactorially inherited disease is distributed normally, with most individuals clustering around a central (mean) measurement and with relatively few individuals located at the extreme tails of the curve. Those at the low (left) end of the curve are unusually resistant to the illness, whereas those at the high (right) end of the curve are unusually susceptible or vulnerable to the disorder. When the total effect of those genes which contribute to the disease, together with the environmental variables impinging upon the individual's genetic potential exceed the threshold level of intensity, those individuals will decompensate and become overtly ill.

(Figure 5). In many or perhaps even most cases, these illnesses tend to be either present or absent, yet they do not show a simple inheritance pattern or chromosomal abnormalities. Nevertheless, epidemiological studies reveal that the intra-familial distributions of these disorders cannot be accounted for solely on the basis of environmental or psychosocial circumstances. Rather, a variety of clear biological *and* environmental factors are involved in the genesis of these diseases. Whenever the sum total of all these genetic and environmental factors exceed a certain *threshold,* the individual's capacity to function and cope breaks down, he decompensates organically, psychiatrically, or both, and becomes incapacitated (see Figure 5). In fact, the threshold between compensation and decompensation is rarely sharply defined and it is more accurate to speak of a more diffuse *threshold area* in which additional environmental factors increase the individual's likelihood of becoming ill (Vogel and Motulsky 1979). We therefore are speaking in terms of a *liability* to decompensate—that is, a graded continuum of increasing susceptibility to becoming ill.

Polygenic inheritance thus involves cumulative contributions from a number of genes which produce only small effects by themselves. These genes may be dominant, recessive, or additive, and they may act to modify the effects of a major gene or to suppress it altogether. Multifactorial inheritance includes traits that arise in response to both polygenic and environmental factors. The incidence of such traits within a population may follow a normal distribution as in the case of body height or intelligence, or follow a discontinuous distribution, being either present or absent as in the case of alcoholism, schizophrenia or diabetes. Liability to decompensation is a graded continum that is normally distributed. However, there is a threshold to this liability below which few or no individuals decompensate and above which most or all individuals are affected.

It can be shown (see Vogel and Motulsky 1979) that if the *concordance* (existence of a trait in both members of a twin pair) of a trait in *monozygotic* (deriving from one egg—i.e., identical) twins is more than four times higher than in *dizygotic* (deriving from two different eggs—i.e., fraternal) twins, then a multifactorial inheritance model with a threshold effect is favored over a simple diallelic model (one involving just two alleles). The converse is not true; a concordance ratio less than four does not rule out a multifactorial model. The twin concordance rates expected to occur with various modes of inheritance are:

Mode of Inheritance	Monozygotic Twin Concordance	Dizygotic Twin Concordance
Autosomal-dominant inheritance	100%	50%
Autosomal-recessive inheritance	100%	25%
Multifactorial inheritance with en-environmental influences (threshold)	40%-60%	4%-8%

(From Table 3.21 in Vogel and Motulsky 1979: 158)

There is evidence that multifactorial inheritance systems may involve a general predisposition leading to a group of related diseases. This appears to be the case with three atopic diseases: atopic dermatitis, bronchial asthma and hay fever. This may also play a role in the case of depressive spectrum disorder, alcoholism and socipathy. Multifactorial inheritance paradigms involve many unspecified genes operating together with environmental factors in the etiology of these disorders. The number of genes is generally thought to be relatively large and the contribution each makes to the overall picture is small. The genes are also thought to act in an additive fashion. When the disease presents as a discontinous and bimodal grouping of "normals" and "affected" individuals, a threshold effect is usually assumed. When the number of genes operating within the context of a specific set of environmental variables falls above the threshold, the individual becomes ill. It has been suggested (Vogel and Motulsky 1979) that one or a few *major genes* may actually play an important role in the genesis of multifactorial disorders. These few major genes may act upon the overall genetic background produced by the various polygenes, and the polygenes may act as modifier genes relative to the major genes. Multifactorial inheritance is summarized in Figures 6 and 7.

Among environmental and random factors, the presence of other coexisting trauma or impairment provides yet another dimension to the development of multifactorial disorders. The more stressed an organism is any one sphere of existence the more likely it is to succumb to pressures from other directions. An organism experiencing severe hypothermia is less resistant to bacterial and viral infection, for example. Conversely, an organism laid low by illness and fever is less resistant to cold or other adverse conditions. Given a genetic substrate which predisposes an individual to alcoholism or any other psychiatric condition, a combination of trauma and decompensation in other areas of life can be sufficient to precipitate the psychiatric illness. For example, the real or symbolic loss of a parent figure is a common experience in both the substance abuse disorders and in depression. It may be that absent such trauma during a vulnerable stage of life, some addicted or depressed individuals might not have decompensated into overt psychiatric illness.

Before discussing the results of genetic studies on alcohol abuse and alcoholism, one important caveat must be stressed: *similar or identical phenotypes are often caused by a variety of geneotypes* (Vogel and Motulsky 1979)! Many superficially or even clinically indistinguishable psychiatric and organic diseases may actually have multiple or heterogeneous etiologies, which often makes the problem of differential diagnosis very difficult.

Are the schizophreniform disorders merely variants of one major underlying disease, for example, or do they represent several different illnesses with similar clinical appearances? Are the differences in expression, severity, and prognosis between early-onset, process schizophrenia and late-onset, so-called acute or "reactive" schizophrenia primarily of kind or degree? Do the affective disorders represent variants of one underlying disorder or are distinct clinical entities with differing etiologies? And is there a real, fundamental difference between "alcoholism," alcohol "abuse" and "problem drinking"? Is the distinction between "primary" and "secondary" alcoholism (see Light 1985) a real one or an

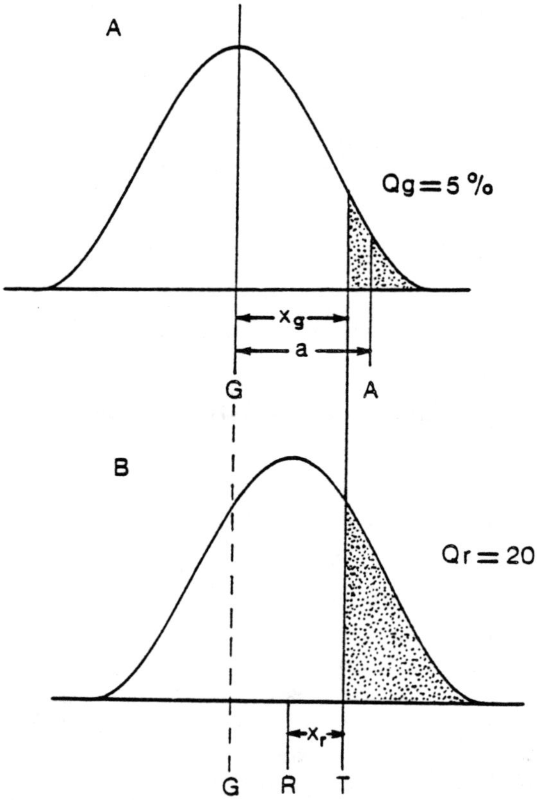

Figure 6. Inheritance of Liability to Disease. All individuals with a combined genetic and environmental load (x-value) greater than the threshold value (T) will express the trait. When the liability to a certain disease in the general population (distribution A) is compared to the liability exhibited by the biological relatives of those affected (distribution B), it can be seen that the mean in distribution B is shifted toward the threshold value. This implies the existence of a genetic component in the development of the illness. The difference between the means of the two distributions (R-G) represents the gain in liability realized when relatives of afflicted patients are selected from the general population. When an illness has an all-or-nothing character, that is, it is either present or it is not, it is assumed that there is an underlying continuum of liability. Below a certain value of liability—the threshold value—the individual has a normal phenotype; above that value he or she is affected with the disease. Whether or not an individual exceeds the threshold value of liability for an illness depends upon his or her genetic susceptibility and the entire set of contributing environmental circumstances. Qg = the incidence of the disease in the general population; Qr = the incidence of the disease among the relatives of affected probands. After Ehrman and Parsons 1976.

artifact of psychiatric nosology and cultural bias? There is abundant evidence to support a variety of interpretations relative to most of these disorders. We simply do not know. And even if these disorders do represent several different illnesses with somewhat different causes, does it make

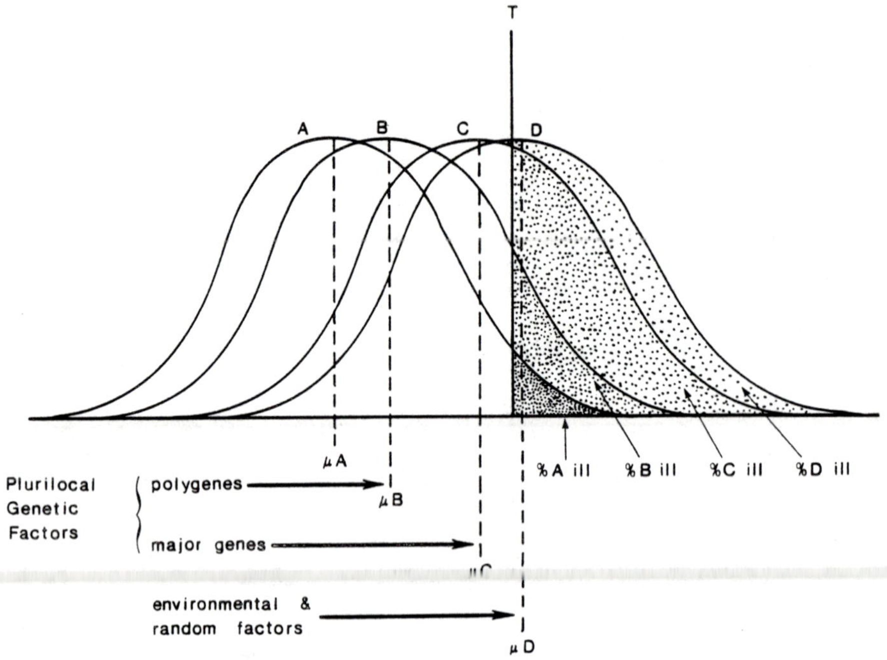

Figure 7. Conceptual Model for Multifactorial Inheritance. Four different curves representing four differing liabilities of susceptibility to a multifactorially inherited disorder; μA = the statistical mean of population A, μB = that of population B, and so forth; T = the threshold value for liability above which the disease is manifested in the phenotype. Population A represents the liability to the disease existing in the population at large—the percentage of population falling ill is shown by the darkest stippling under the far right portion of curve A. The presence of polygenic factors predisposing to the disorder is shown by curve B; the mean is shifted to the right toward the threshold value, and a higher proportion of this population is affected by the illness (moderately dark stippling). One or a few major genes acting upon predisposing genetic background in population C may significantly enhance the liability to illness so that a large percentage are affected (moderately light stippling). Environmental factors acting upon a strongly genetically predisposed population may shift the liability so far to the right that the mean liability actually lies above the threshold (μD), and most of the population falls ill (lightest stippling).

any difference? We do not know. In most cases, psychiatric disorders behave as if they were representative of both the single-disease and the heterogeneously-caused models.

Genetic Factors in Alcoholism

It has long been observed that alcoholism runs in families, and many authorities have believed that it had strong genetic or hereditary underpinnings. A major problem, of course, has been how to differentiate between biological factors and sociocultural and environmental factors, which also tend to run in families. Is the alcoholism in the son of an alcoholic father due to heredity or is it more the result of growing up in an alcoholic environment characterized by severe family disruption and discord, and an abusive and often absent, inconsistent parent? A number of early and rather unsophisticated studies indicated that the male relatives of alcoholics have alcoholism rates themselves of 25 to 50 percent, and that the rate for female relatives is five to eight percent. This represents a rate for both sexes of nearly five times that actually seen in the general population (Goodwin 1976).

In a benchmark study, an American psychiatrist and his American and Danish colleagues compared the biological sons of alcoholic parents who were adopted into foster homes in infancy with a similarly adopted control group of biological sons of nonalcoholic parents (Goodwin *et al.* 1973). In an extension of this research, this team also compared the drinking problems in adopted biological sons of alcoholics with their nonadopted brothers raised by the alcoholic parent (Goodwin *et al.* 1974). These two studies provide compelling evidence that severe alcoholism, at least, is under much stronger genetic than environmental influence. This and other evidence is reviewed in a popular book by the senior author of these two papers (Goodwin 1976), and the reader is referred there for further explanation and details.

These investigators selected their subjects from a pool of about 5,000 cases of adoption in and around Copenhagen from 1924 through 1947. In order to evaluate the role played by inheritance, a *proband* group of adopted men who had at least one biological alcoholic parent was compared with a *control* group of adopted men, neither of whose biological parents were alcoholic. The biological parents were diagnosed as alcoholic on the basis of one or more hospitalizations for alcoholism. All subjects in both groups were adopted into foster homes in early infancy and were therefore not "contaminated" (for purposes of the study) by the alcoholic environment of their biological families. The criminal records of all adoptees and their biological parents, if any, were also included in the study. About 85 percent of the alcoholic parents of the probands were fathers. The biological families of the adopted control group differed from those of the proband group only in that neither of the parents had ever been hospitalized for alcoholism. The adoptive families for both groups were similar in all respects; there was a slightly greater incidence of depression among the foster-mothers of the probands than in the case of controls and a slightly greater incidence of alcoholism among the foster-fathers of the controls relative to the probands, but neither of the differences were statistically significant.[25] The socioeconomic and educational levels of the probands and controls were similar, and the average age of both was 30 and the age-range 23 to 45 years at the time of the study.

If environmental factors do play a significant role in the etiology of alcoholism we would expect the rates of alcoholism to be similar in both the probands and controls. In fact, the probands *showed four times the rate of alcoholism as the controls,* strongly suggesting that heredity is a major factor in the development of this disease. The probands and controls differed significantly from each other only with respect to alcoholism and divorce. Divorce was three times higher in the probands than in the controls. Other than divorces and alcoholism the two groups were statistically indistinguishable, and the incidence of other psychiatric disorders (clinically evident depression, anxiety neurosis, criminality and other drug addiction) was low in both. Interestingly, the higher divorce rate among the probands was not related to drinking; moderate drinkers among the probands were as likely as heavy drinkers and alcoholics to be divorced. The high divorce rate among alcoholics in general may thus not be due solely to the alcoholism itself.

The control group exhibited a slightly higher incidence of heavy and "problem" drinking than did the proband group. As previously noted, the foster-parents of the control groups showed a higher, but statistically insignificant, level of alcoholism, Goodwin (1976, page 74) observed that *"severe forms of alcohol abuse may have a genetic predisposition but that heavy drinking itself, even when responsible for occasional problems, reflects predominantly nongenetic factors"* [italics his]. The criteria for determining the drinking status for the subjects in this study were as follows (Goodwin 1976, page 72):

(1) Moderate drinker—neither a teetotaler nor a heavy drinker.

[25] A statistically significant difference represents an arbitrarily chosen probability value that two measurements being compared could not have occurred by chance. Consider the normal curve in Figure 4. The great majority of measurements cluster about a central mean and the two "tails" of the curve represent those few extreme measurements in either direction above and below the mean contained in the population or sample. Most individuals have rather normal heights within a small range of variation, for example, and only a few persons will be either extremely tall or extremely short. The significance level is arbitrarily set, but convention usually suggests rejection at the five percent *significance level* ($P < 0.05$). In other words, if one measurement has a likelihood of less than five percent of deviating from a measurement against which it is being compared (a measurement in the proband group relative to one in the control group) *on the basis of chance alone*—that is, there is more than a 95 percent chance that these numbers come from different populations, but about a five percent chance that these are just extreme measurement in the same population—then the difference is considered to be statistically significant.

(2) Heavy drinker—drank daily for at least one year and consumed six or more drinks at least two or three times per month or drank six or more drinks at least once a week, but who reported no problems because of drinking.

(3) Problem drinker—meets the criteria for heavy drinker and who has problems resulting from drinking which are insufficient in number and intensity for a diagnosis of alcoholism.

(4) Alcoholic—meets the criteria for a heavy drinker and who has problems in at least three of the following areas:

(a) social disapproval of drinking by friends and relatives; marital discord resulting from drinking.

(b) trouble on the job due to drinking; traffic arrest and other police action because of drinking.

(c) frequent blackouts; tremor; withdrawal hallucinations and/or convulsions; delerium tremens.

(d) loss of control (wanting to stop drinking on any occasion but being unable to do so); morning drinking (repeated morning drinking, not just one or two before-breakfast drinking episodes).

The probands had an average of 2.05 alcohol-related problems as compared with 1.23 among the controls, and the difference was statistically significant. More than 60 percent of the subjects in both groups were still in their twenties at the time of the study. Therefore most had not yet traversed the age of risk for the development of alcoholism (20 to 45). It is not clear whether the incidence of divorce and/or alcoholism will increase or whether the difference between the probands and controls will continue to grow.

As a followup to this study, Goodwin and his colleagues interviewed and evaluated the brothers of adopted probands who had not been adopted out and who were raised by the biological parent(s). Twenty probands had brothers who had been raised by the biological, alcoholic parent, and 30 of these siblings were available for study (Goodwin *et al.* 1974). The interviews were conducted in Danish by a Danish psychiatrist and were "blind" from the start—that is the interviewer had no idea which subjects were born to alcoholic parents and which were not. The results of these interviews were analyzed blind in the United States to avoid any bias. The non-adopted sons differed from their adopted siblings in being, on the average, three years older, less likely to have been married, belonging to a lower social class, and in having parents-of-upbringing with higher rates of alcoholism (by definition, since all of the parents of the non-adopted siblings were alcoholic) and antisocial behavior.

The purpose of the study was to compare blood brothers who had no contact with each other but who had in common an alcoholic biological parent. Because one sibling had been adopted out in early infancy into a foster home and the other(s) were raised by the alcoholic parent, the results of the study should shed additional light on the relative importance of heredity and environmental factors in the development of alcoholism. If environment were to play a significant role, we would expect the siblings raised by the alcoholic parent to show higher rates of alcoholism.

The study's major finding was that the sons of alcoholics were equally likely to become alcoholic regardless of whether they were raised in a nonalcoholic foster home from infancy on or by the alcoholic biological parent! The fact that the non-adopted siblings were generally older and therefore further along into the age-risk for developing alcoholism only strengthens the finding.[26] Furthermore, the family psychopathology of the non-adopted siblings was markedly greater as would be expected in actively alcoholic families. The non-adopted siblings had more disrupted childhood environments than their adopted brothers, more had been on welfare and otherwise had come to the attention of child welfare and social agencies, and more had exhibited truancy, disobedience and poor academic performance in childhood. Although all these factors are associated[27] with an increased risk for alcoholism, the men in this group showed no greater incidence of alcoholism than their adopted-out brothers. In view of the foregoing it is remarkable how little environmental factors appear to contribute to the development of alcoholism.

Other adoption studies either support the foregoing findings (Amark 1951) or are equivocal because of methodological deficiencies (Roe and Burks 1945). The general conclusion appears to be that *only* alcoholism is transmitted genetically irrespective of family environment, whereas mere heavy drinking and problem drinking may derive primarily from psychosocical causes (Goodwin 1976). On the other hand, *"Simply living*

---

[26]The mean age of the adopted sons was 30 years and the range 23 to 45; the mean age of the non-adopted sons was 33 years and the range 20 to 51 (Goodwin *et al.* 1974).

[27]A statistical association or correlation of a trait with certain environmental or individual variables does *not* necessarily indicate a causal relationship. For example, low socioeconomic status is associated with increased psychiatric disturbance of all kinds, including alcoholism, but this may merely reflect a downward social "drift" due to general functional impairment due to these illnesses. Low socioeconomic environments may not therefore actually *cause* these disorders. Higher scores by children on intelligence tests may be positively correlated with physical stature, but being taller does not cause anyone to be more intelligent—it simply reflects greater age, experience and maturity.

with an alcoholic parent appear(s) to have no relationship to the development of alcoholism" (Goodwin *et al.* 1974) [italics theirs]. Still another study (Schuckit *et al.* 1972) indicates that individuals raised apart from one of their biological parents, where either the biological parent or a surrogate step-parent with whom they lived had a drinking problem, were themselves more likely to have a drinking problem if their biological parent from whom they were separated was diagnosed as alcoholic than if their surrogate, but not their biological, parent was alcoholic.

Of 32 alcoholics and non-alcoholics coming mostly from broken homes, 62 percent of the former and only 20 percent of the latter had an alcoholic biological parent. And none of the half-sibs (those with only one biological parent in common) had lived with an alcoholic foster-parent in contrast to five percent of the non-alcoholic half-sibs that had lived with an alcoholic foster-parent. This study also showed that about 50 percent of the half-sibs who shared an alcoholic biological parent were themselves alcoholic regardless of whether they were raised by an alcoholic (either biological or adopted) or a non-alcoholic parent. Few of the half-sibs with non-alcoholic biological parents were themselves alcoholic, although twice as many (14% as compared to 8%) became alcoholic if one of the rearing parents was alcoholic. The authors noted that having an alcoholic biological parent was the only consistent predictor of alcoholism in half-siblings. They suggested that persons with an alcoholic parent inherit a *genetic load,* that is, a liability-threshold susceptibility to developing alcoholism.

A study in Sweden (Kaij 1960) compared 58 monozygotic with 138 dizygotic twin-pairs in which at least one twin pair was documented as alcoholic by one of two County Temperance Board registries. Of these, 31 MZ pairs (53%) showed perfect concordance relative to the severity of alcoholism as compared to 70 DZ pairs (28%); the difference was statistically significant. Moreover, in the DZ pairs the concordance increased as the severity of alcoholism increased, which was not true of the DZ pairs. Interestingly, social and intellectual deterioration presumably due to alcohol abuse was more closely correlated with zygosity than with the severity of drinking, whether the twins were identical or fraternal. Thus, a severely alcoholic, deteriorated MZ twin was more likely to have a more moderate-drinking twin with deterioration than was a deteriorated DZ twin. It may be that alcoholism and alcoholic deterioration are inherited independently of each other. Several psychiatrists were involved in rating each individual in the study and interrater agreement was high.

In a study in Finland, Partanen *et al.* (1966) employed 172 MZ and 557 same-sexed DZ twins born between 1920 and 1929. The ages of these subjects at the time of the study was 28 to 37. They found no differences between MZ and DZ twins with regard to the consequences of drinking, but frequency and amount of drinking as well as abstinence were all more concordant in MZ than DZ twins. Three identifiable factors appeared from the study: frequency of drinking per unit time, amount consumed and lack of control, all with fairly high *heritability* values.[28] The heritability for lack of control was higher in younger twins but not in older ones, presumably reflecting a greater severity of alcoholism in the former.

Still another group of investigators in Des Moines, Iowa compared male adoptees with first-degree alcoholic relatives (biological mother or father) with adoptees having second-degree alcoholic relatives (brothers or sisters of biological parents or biological grandparents) and a control group of adoptees whose biological relatives had other psychiatric diagnoses than alcoholism or else none at all. (Cadoret *et al.* 1980.) As in the other such studies described here, these men were adopted into foster families at a very early age and contact with the biological relatives was minimal. The adoptees were also matched on age, time spent in foster care and the age of the biological mother at the time of the adoptee's birth. The purpose of this investigation was to evaluate the relative importance of biological background, environmental factors, and the interaction, if any, between the two variables in the development of alcoholism in the adoptees. The environmental factors examined included any existing psychiatric or behavior disturbance in the adoptive home, including alcoholism, and the effect of "discontinuous mothering" due to pre-adoption institutional care. A multiple statistical regression model of the following type was employed:

---

[28]Heritability, here used in the narrow sense, is an indicator of the predictability of an individual's phenotype based upon the known phenotypes of his close relatives. It is usually defined as some variation of $h^2 = Vg/Vp$, where Vg = the genotypic variance and Vp = the phenotypic variance; h^2 thus is the ratio of the genetic variance to the phenotypic variance. The higher the value of h^2 the greater is the genetic component of the phenotype. The *variance* of a population or sample is equal to the square of the standard deviation (Figure 4). It is the second total moment about the mean, that is the sum of the squared deviations

$$\left[\sum_{i=1}^{n} (X_i - \bar{x})^2 \right]$$

from the mean divided by the number of measurements in the population or sample. Whereas the mean, or first total moment about the mean, is a measure of central tendency, the variance is a measure of the variability. (See also footnote 40).

log [odds in favor of adoptee alcoholism] = [biological background + environmental predictors].

A hierarchical analysis of multiway interactions between all the independent variables examined was conducted. From an original model that included all possible interactions (e.g., simultaneous existence of first-degree alcoholic biological relatives, significant discontinuous mothering experience, and psychiatric disorder in the adoptive family constitutes a 3-way interaction), those variables that were not statistically significant were rejected, and the remaining model interpreted.

A significant association between having first- and/or second-degree alcoholic biological relatives and alcoholism in the adoptees was obtained. There was also a non-significant association between a history of childhood conduct disorder and alcoholism in the adoptees, although acceptance of the null hypothesis was close ($P = 0.0561$).[29] There was no indication that environmental variables played any role in the development of alcoholism in these subjects. The authors concluded:

> 1. In this sample the environmental variables, taken together, explain less [about the development of alcoholism in the adoptees] than the biological predictors taken alone.
> 2. In this sample when the environmental variables are added to the biologic background variables, prediction of adoptee alcoholism does not improve.
> 3. In this sample there is no evidence that environmental variables interact significantly with biologic variables, to potentiate or ameliorate the risks of adoptee alcoholism due to biologic background.

Although several adoptive families had an alcoholic member there was no alcoholism in any adoptee from these families, further supporting the lack of any environmental effect. There was also no relationship between psychiatric disturbance of any kind, including alcoholism, in the adoptive family and alcoholism in the adoptee. Because the authors considered the association between childhood conduct disorder and adoptee alcoholism to be significant, they looked into the biological backgrounds of these adoptees who were psychiatrically diagnosed as

[29]In any statistical test of significance the null hypothesis being tested states that there is *no* significant difference between the samples being compared. If the probability value associated with the test is less than five percent ($P < 0.05$), the interpretation is that there is less than a five percent likelihood that the differences observed could be due to chance alone *(although this could be that time and the rejection of the null hypothesis would be wrong!)*. The null hypothesis is then rejected and the alternative hypothesis, that there *is* a difference between the samples is accepted. In the above case the null hypothesis should barely be accepted (although the authors considered the association to be significant).

being both alcoholic and sociopathic. There was no evidence that an alcoholic biological background was a predictor to antisocial personality or that alcoholism in these individuals was secondary to sociopathy. Although exposure of the adoptee to discontinuous mothering was associated with adoptee antisocial behavior in adolescence, it was not associated with adoptee alcoholism. Finally, no association between the socioeconomic status of the adopted family and adoptee alcoholism was found. [But see below.]

The most intriguing of the adoptee studies relative to alcoholism was recently carried out in Sweden in a collaboration of American and Swedish investigators (Cloninger *et al.*, 1981). These collaborators distinguished two forms of alcoholism with distinct genetic and environmental causes and differing expressions in men and association with criminal behavior and sociopathy. These authors suggested that susceptibility to alcoholism derived neither entirely from genetic nor entirely from environmental factors, nor from simply the sum of separate genetic and environmental contributions. Rather, they suggested, specific combinations of predisposing genetic influences and environmental "stressors" must interact in order for alcoholism to develop in most cases.

These investigators studied a sample of 862 men born out of wedlock in Stockholm from 1930 through 1949 who were adopted prior to age three by biologically unrelated foster parents. These adopted men ranged in age from 23 to 43 years at the time of the study, but age differences appeared to have no effect on the risk for alcoholism in these subjects. Detailed information about the adoptees and their biological adopted families was available from a number of sources, including child welfare agencies, registrations for alcohol abuse by the Temperance Board,[30] criminal conviction registrations, and medical and occupational information recorded by agencies of the National Health Insurance. Alcohol abuse among the adoptees was categorized according to severity rather than mere presence or absence. The authors addressed the following questions in their study: (1) What characteristics in the biological parents influence the risk of alcohol abuse in adoptees? (2) What characteristics of the adopted parents and the adoptive environment influence the risk of alcohol abuse in adoptees? (3) How do genetic and environmental determinants interact to produce alcohol abuse?

[30]In Sweden, a Temperance Board in each community registers persons guilty of intoxication or intemperance, and has the duty and authority to impose fines and to mandate and supervise alcoholism reeducation, treatment and rehabilitation, and when they deem necessary, impose mandatory hospitalization.

A complex series of statsitical protocals was employed to identify the background variables associated with the risk of alcohol abuse in these subjects, and all correlations were considered significant only if their probability of occurring by chance alone was less than five percent. Of the 862 adoptees, 151 or 17.5 percent had some record of alcohol abuse: 64 or 7.4 percent had one Temperance Board registration and were labelled as *mild abusers*; another 36 men or 4.2 percent had two or three registrations and were labelled as *moderate abusers*; and another 51 of these men had four or more registrations, compulsory treatment for alcoholism or hospitalization with a diagnosis of alcoholism. The remaining 711 adoptees appeared to be nonabusers.

The biological fathers of mild abusers had recurrent alcohol abuse not requiring treatment and they exhibited little criminality and had higher socioeconomic status than the fathers of the other abusers. The biological mothers of these men were also frequently alcohol abusers.

The biological fathers of moderate alcohol abusers had histories of recurrent alcohol abuse, low socioeconomic status and a high level of criminal convictions. The criminal and alcoholic behavior of these fathers often began in adolescence. The biological mothers of moderate alcohol abusing adoptees were generally similar to the mothers of non-alcoholics.

The biological parents of severe abusers were in general similar to those of mild alcohol abusers, except that the fathers of these men had the lowest socioeconomic and occupational status of any group.

It was further found that the 239 adoptees who remained with their biological mothers beyond age six months a risk for later alcohol abuse 1.5 times greater than the others (23% as compared with 16%, respectively; $P<0.001$).[31] The only significant variable about the adoptive parents relative to alcohol abuse among the adoptees was low occupational status. Alcoholism in the adoptive families did *not* increase the risk of alcohol abuse in the adoptees. On the contrary, alcohol abuse among the adoptees raised in alcoholic foster homes showed a non-significant *decrease* relative to those reared in non-alcoholic foster homes (13% as contrasted with 18%).

Other than low occupational status of the adoptive father, extensive institutional care prior to adoptive placement was the only environmental

[31]That is, a probability of 0.1 percent. This means there is less than one-tenth of one percent likelihood that the difference between these two groups was due to chance alone. Stated otherwise, it is more than 99.9 percent likely that the results represent a real difference between the two groups. This level of rejection of the null hypothesis is referred to as being *very highly significant*.

factor associated with increased risk for alcohol abuse. These two factors characterized both mild and severe alcohol abuse, but to a smaller extent in the case of mild abusers.

The increase in mild alcohol abuse was four times greater among those adoptees having both genetic and environmental predisposing factors in their background over those with neither. Genetic factors alone appeared to be significant in the etiology of moderate alcohol abuse, and the risk increased nine times in genetically predisposed adoptees regardless of their environmental backgrounds. In the case of severe alcohol abuse, small increases in risk were noted from either genetic or environmental background, but neither was significant and there was no interaction between heredity and environment. The genetic variables underlying the development of both mild and severe alcohol abuse were similar, as previously noted, *except for the occupational status of the biological parents.*

The authors noted the distinct genetic overlap between mild and severe alcohol abuse and suggested that the presence or absence of specific environmental influences will largely determine the severity of abuse in a given individual with this genetic predisposition. Those individuals who are genetically predisposed to either mild or severe alcohol abuse who also have a biological or adoptive parent with low occupational status and/or experienced prolonged preplacement institutional care *will show an increased risk only for severe abuse.* The predisposition to severe abuse thus has two components: (1) a genetic component that is the same as for mild abuse, and (2) a predisposition to low occupational status from either hereditary (the biological parent) or postnatal (the adoptive parent) sources. When adoptees with a genetic tendency to severe abuse (alcoholic biological parent with low occupational status) were placed in an adoptive family predisposing to mild abuse (adoptive parent with high occupational status), there was an increased risk for both mild and severe abuse. In the main, the expression of mild or severe abuse was determined largely by the postnatal situation, and only to a lesser extent by the socioeconomic status of the biological parents.

These investigators suggested that there are two distinct types of alcohol abuse with differing genetic and environmental underpinnings. The less common type, moderate alcohol abuse, appears to be determined solely by genetic traits deriving from the adoptee's biological father. This type of alcohol abuser is associated with a high level of criminal behavior by the biological fathers and it accounts for about 24 percent of the alcohol abuse by adoptees. These authors did not report on the presence or absence of criminal behavior in the adoptees themselves. It cannot be determined then whether antisocial traits in the fathers were passed on to their biological sons. Recent evidence is compelling, however, that such behavior is genetically inherited (see below).

The other type of liability to alcohol abuse produces both mild and severe abuse; it is much more common and accounts for about 76 percent of all abuse by the adoptees. This category of alcohol abuse is strongly influenced by postnatal environmental parameters, specifically the socioeconomic status of the adoptive parents and the degree of preplacement institutionalization experienced by the adoptee. This type of alcoholism, termed *milieu-limited* (as contrasted with *male-limited*) is associated with alcoholism without criminality in the biological parents. Both parents frequently contribute to their offsprings' alcohol abuse in milieu-limited alcohol abuse, quite unlike the case in male-limited alcoholism.

These two types of alcoholism resemble in many respects what others have referred to as *primary* or *essential* ("garden-variety") alcoholism and *secondary* or *reactive* alcoholism. Primary or uncomplicated alcoholics comprise the vast majority of alcoholics. They usually present no other major psychiatric disturbance in the absence of significant organic brain damage from their drinking and they do not tend to have significant criminal records outside of alcohol-related traffic offenses and other misdemeanors. They have little real criminal or sociopathic involvement otherwise. Secondary alcoholism is thought to develop because of a previously existing other psychiatric disorder such as schizophrenia, bipolar disorder or most especially, sociopathy,[32] About one-fifth of all male alcoholics are in fact also sociopaths, which closely approximates the percentage of male-limited alcoholics in the study by Cloninger and his colleagues. If there is a relationship between these several diagnostic entities, then sociopathic-type (male-limited) alcoholism ironically appears to constitute a more fundamentally "primary" type of alcohol abuse, since it appears to be in no way influenced by environmental factors. "Garden-variety" or milieu-limited alcoholism would then appear to be more "reactive" in the sense of responding at least partly to environmental stressors.

[32]I have never been convinced that the type of alcohol abuse seen in schizophrenics and some manic patients represents true *alcoholism* as it exists in primary alcoholics and sociopathic "secondary" alcoholics.

Finally, a comment must be made about the various disparities in the adoption studies conducted to date. Goodwin and his colleagues found that environmental parameters contributed very little if anything to the development of alcoholism among their subjects. I don't agree with the suggestion by Cloninger and colleagues that the Danish adoptees can all be referred to the male-limited type of alcoholism simply because environmental factors were found not to be important. It is simply asking too much to consider that such a large sample could consist almost totally of sociopathic alcoholics. And the fascinating results of the Swedish study must be contrasted with the Des Moines study which specifically looked at the relationship between alcoholism and socioeconomic status of the adoptive parents. In Sweden this was found to be a significant factor; in Iowa it was not.

It may be that different ethnic populations exhibit differing subtypes of alcohol abuse, and that the several studies reflected just that. The type of florid alcoholism seen in the great majority of Native Americans is certainly quantitatively and *qualitatively* different from that seen in American whites or blacks. A great deal more work needs to be accomplished before we can begin to sift out the various contributions of all the genetic and environmental variables. And adoption studies will continue to be one of our most useful methodologies to this end. What is clear is that heredity and genetic factors play the major role in the predisposition toward alcohol abuse, and that environmental factors, when they do exert an effect, act only to modify these underlying biological susceptibilities.

Several cross-fostering studies conducted quite independently of the studies on alcoholism (although in some cases the same pool of adoptees was used) have provided compelling evidence that criminal behavior and sociopathy are genetically inherited. Adoptees of non-criminal biological fathers reared in a criminal foster home have the same rates of criminality as those lacking criminality in either the biological or the foster parents (Horn 1978). In other words, without a genetic predisposition to criminal behavior, environment seems to have no significant effect. Sons of criminal biological fathers raised in a non-criminal foster environment are twice as likely to be criminals as controls. Adoptees having criminal biological parents who were also raised in a criminal foster home showed three times the rate of criminality as controls, showing that environment can enhance a criminal predisposition. Several studies in several European countries and in the United States all showed greater concordance for criminality among monozygotic than dizygotic twins—some of them very considerably higher (Vogel and Motulsky 1979). More recently, a study of 14,427 adoptees in an unnamed European country showed a statistically significant correlation between the adoptees and their biological parents relative to criminal convictions. This was especially true in the case of chronic and recidivist criminality. No environmental variables could satisfactorily explain this relationship and the evidence implies that strong biological predisposing factors are involved in the etiology of at least some criminal behavior (Mednik *et al.* 1984). This lends support to the hypothesis proposed by Cloninger and his colleagues relative to milieu-limited and male-limited alcoholism—that is, that criminality has a strong genetic component.

Several biological studies relative to the etiology have focused upon alcohol metabolism. Monozygotic twins were found to have high concordance for rates of alcohol metabolism, with mean intrapair differences for MZ twins being 0.004 mg/ml/hour as compared with mean intrapair differences of 0.05 mg/ml/hour (Vogel and Motulsky 1979). These values differ by a factor of more than 12, and computed heritability values suggest nearly exclusive genetic control of this parameter. About 85 percent of Japanese persons have an atypical alcohol dehydrogenase in their livers; 15 percent of Japanese have the "normal" type of enzyme found in most Europeans. The atypical enzyme metabolizes alcohol more rapidly than the normal type, and thus produces higher levels of acetaldehyde. Because the excess of acetaldehyde cannot be cleared from the body by aldehyde dehydrogenase as rapidly as it builds up, toxic levels are thought to accumulate and precipitate the characteristic "flushing" response to alcohol exhibited by many Japanese. The flushing syndrome also typically includes abdominal discomfort, muscle weakness, dizziness, rapid pulse and a fall in blood pressure (hypotension). This flushing response is present from infancy, showing that it cannot be a learned response. In contrast to Orientals, only 34 percent of white adults exhibit this flushing response to a test challenge. It has been suggested by a number of authors that this aversive response to moderate doses of alcohol may underlie the low vulnerability to alcoholism thought to characterize Oriental people. These individuals are thought to be prone to drink less because of their unpleasant response to the drug. There is some evidence, however, that alcoholics may be increasing in Japan, although this is mainly anecdotal (Mendelson and Mello 1979).

Studies on Native Americans have produced conflicting results (Mendelson and Mello 1979). Native Americans are notorious for their extreme rates of florid alcoholism. Some Indians and Inuits (Eskimos) metabolize alcohol more slowly than whites after equivalent doses. However Ojibwas (Chippewas) metabolize it more rapidly than do whites or Chinese, and Chinese metabolize alcohol faster than do whites (presumably because of the atypical alcohol dehydrogenase). Thus, various Native American tribes with extreme rates of alcoholism metabolize alcohol both more rapidly and more slowly than do white controls. It is therefore not possible to correlate rates of alcohol clearance with risk for alcoholism (Mendelson and Mello 1979).[33]

The oxidation of large amounts of ethanol *in vivo* can interfere with the normal metabolic breakdown of neurotransmitters in the brain. Dopamine and norepinephrine are converted into their respective aldehyde derivatives by the enzymes monoamine oxidase (MAO) and catechole-O-methyltransferase (COMT). Similarly, serotonin (5-hydroxytryptamine) is converted into its aldehyde metabolite, 5-hydroxyindole-3-acetaldehyde, by MAO and 5-hydroxyindole-O-methyltransferase (5-HIOMT). These aminealdehydes are normally then either (1) reduced into their respective alcohols by alcohol dehydrogenase, accompanied by the oxidation of NADH plus H^+ into NAD^+, or (2) they are oxidized into their derivative acids by aldehyde dehydrogenase, accompanied by the reduction of NAD^+ into NADH and H^+ (Figure 8; see also Light 1986a for a complete discussion of this).

The metabolic pathway for alcohol oxidation, most of which occurs in the liver, is:

$$(1)\quad \underset{\text{ethanol}}{CH_3CH_2OH + NAD^+} \xrightarrow[\text{DEHYDROGENASE}]{\text{ALCOHOL}} \underset{\text{acetaldehyde}}{CH_3CHO} + NADH + H^+$$

$$(2)\quad \underset{\text{acetaldehyde}}{CH_3CHO} + NAD^+ \xrightarrow[\text{DEHYDROGENASE}]{\text{ALDEHYDE}} \underset{\text{acetate}}{CH_3COOH} + NADH + H^+$$

The mass effect of large amounts of acetaldehyde resulting from ethanol oxidation outcompetes the aminealdehydes for the enzyme alcohol dehydrogenase (Figure 8), thereby blocking the conversion of the aminealdehyde into its acid derivative. The pathway is therefore shifted to favor the conversion of the aminealdehyde into its derivative alcohol. The excess hydrogen or reducing equivalents (NADH and H^+) generated

[33]Both Indians and whites with a history of heavy drinking metabolize alcohol more rapidly than controls, presumably due to the induction of microsomal enzymes (see Light 1985).

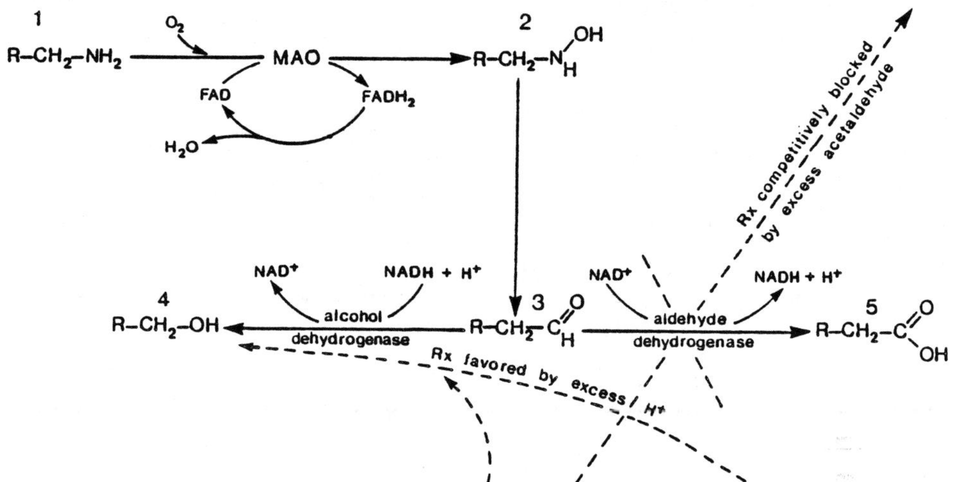

Figure 8. Inhibition of Monoamine Metabolism by Ethanol. Monoamine oxidase catalyzes the oxidative deamination of catecholeamines and other amines in a process in which FAD (a flavoprotein molecule involved in electron transport) is reduced to $FADH_2$ and oxygen is absorbed and a water molecule given off. The amine precursor (1) is first converted into its intermediate hydroxylamine (2). The intermediate is then converted into an aldehyde (3), a transient metabolite which then undergoes one of two reactions: (a) oxidation by aldehyde dehydrogenase into its acid (5) or (b) reduction by alcohol dehydrogenase into its alcohol (4). When large amounts of ethanol are metabolized, the mass effect of the resulting acetaldehyde (7) outcompetes the aminealdehyde for the enzyme aldehyde dehydrogenase, and blocks the conversion of that amine metabolite into its acid form [8 = acetate]. The generation of excess reducing equivalents [NADH and H^+] consequent to ethanol and acetaldehyde oxidation compounds the inhibition of aminealdehyde oxidation, and also favors its reduction into the alcohol form. But because of the competition between ethanol and the aminealdehyde for alcohol dehydrogenase, there is a net buildup of both the aminealdehyde and acetaldehyde. Both aldehydes can then form condensation products with naturally occurring catecholeamine and indoleamine neurotransmitters (see also Figure 9). From Light 1986a, Figure 26.

by ethanol and acetaldehyde oxidation (see Light 1985 for a detailed discussion of this) also inhibit the oxidation of the aminealdehyde into its acid, and favor its reduction into the alcohol. However, the high concentration of ethyl alcohol competitively excludes the aminealdehyde from alcohol dehydrogenase (Figure 8). There is thus a net buildup of both aminealdehydes and acetaldehyde (many studies have consistently shown that alcoholics exhibit higher concentrations of acetaldehyde following alcohol intake than do nonalcoholics). Both of these aldehydes could conceivably then form non-enzymatic condensation products with endogenous catecholamines (particularly dopamine) and indolealkylamines such as tryptophan and serotonin (Figure 9).

Such condensation products are known to form irreversible, heterocyclic compounds at least *in vitro* (Figure 9). If the starting amine-compound is a catecholamine such as dopamine, the condensation products formed will be *tetrahydroisoquinolines* (THIQ's). If the starting amine-compound are indolealkylamines such as tryptophan or its neurotransmitter derivative, serotonin, the condensation products will be *tetrahydro-beta-carbolines* (THBC's). Dopamine and acetaldehyde generated by ethanol oxidation condense to form *salsolinol* (Figure 9), which may then act as a false neurotransmitter in central catacholaminergic neurons. More importantly, dopamine and its own aldehyde metabolite can condense to form *tetrahydropapaveroline* (THPV), a potent beta-adrenoreceptor agonist. THPV is also a precursor molecule in the biosynthetic pathway for morphine and other opiate alkaloids in the opium poppy. THPV may occur in dopamine-rich regions of the brain consequent to the oxidation of large amounts of ethanol. A number of investigators have suggested that an opiate-like physical dependence involving the endogenous opioid (enkephalin) receptors may be one of the consequences of prolonged alcohol abuse (Davis and Walsh 1970; Myers and Critcher 1982; Summer 1985; Myers 1985).

Studies of the pharmacological effects of these aminealdehyde products have consistently shown that salsolinol, THPV and THBC produce exaggerated voluntary ethanol consumption patterns in strains of laboratory rodents which are normally alcohol-aversive (Melchior and Myers 1976; Myers and Melchior 1977; Cohen 1979; Melchior 1980; Myers 1985). Moreover these abnormal drinking behaviors are extraordinarily long-lasting, if indeed not permanent, following 8 to 12 days of intraventricular infusion of aldehyde adducts into the brains of these animals. Rats will self-infuse both acetaldehyde and salsolinol intracerebrally, leading some investigators to suggest that these substances have reinforcing properties (see Hirst *et al.* 1985). Very high doses of THIQ's infused into the cerebral ventricles of alcohol-depdendent mice appear to increase the severity of ethanol withdrawal (Blume *et al.* 1976).

Salsolinol has been found in brain tissue of animals given ethanol as well as compounds which inhibit dopamine and/or acetaldehyde breakdown, although other workers were unable to detect it in animals given ethanol alone (Hirst *et al.* 1985). Sjöquist and her colleagues (1982)

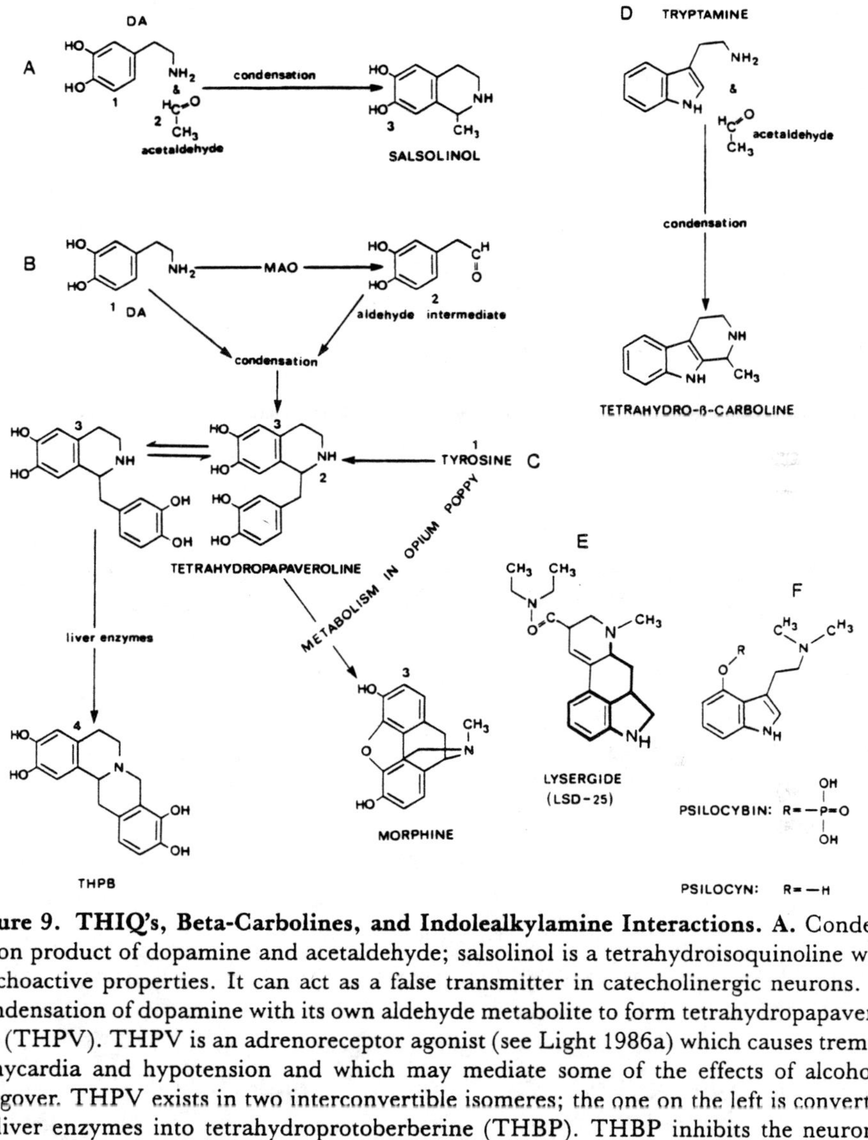

Figure 9. THIQ's, Beta-Carbolines, and Indolealkylamine Interactions. A. Condensation product of dopamine and acetaldehyde; salsolinol is a tetrahydroisoquinoline with psychoactive properties. It can act as a false transmitter in catecholinergic neurons. **B.** Condensation of dopamine with its own aldehyde metabolite to form tetrahydropapaveroline (THPV). THPV is an adrenoreceptor agonist (see Light 1986a) which causes tremor, tachycardia and hypotension and which may mediate some of the effects of alcoholic hangover. THPV exists in two interconvertible isomeres; the one on the left is converted by liver enzymes into tetrahydroprotoberberine (THBP). THBP inhibits the neuronal uptake of Ca^{2+} and depresses the activity of ATPases (see Light 1986a); it also interacts directly with dopaminergic receptors. **C.** The pathway by which morphine is naturally synthesized in the opium poppy. THPV is an intermediate step, and a similar conversion may occur in dopamine-rich regions of the brain. **D.** Condensation of tryptophan (and also of serotonin) with acetaldehyde to form psychoactive tetrahydro-beta-carbolines. **E.** LSD-25: the heavy lines outline the serotonin skeleton. **F.** Psilocybin and psilocyn: the indolealkylamine skeleton is obvious. Tetrahydro-β-carbolines, lysergide and the psilocybinlike compounds produce their psychoactive effects by interacting with serotonin receptors in the brain. The numbers indicate the sequence of reactions in pathways B and C. From Light 1986a, Figure 27.

detected salsolinol in the striatum and other limbic areas of rats chronically exposed to alcohol, as well as in controls. It has also been reported from the urine and cerebrospinal fluid of both alcoholic and non-alcoholic human subjects; however, salsolinol levels did not change following ethanol administration, although alcoholics exhibited higher urine levels than did non-alcoholics (Sjöquist *et al.* 1981). Other workers have also reported that alcoholics excrete significantly higher levels of dopamine-derived THIQ's than do non-alcoholics.

Recently, Sjöquist (1985) found a very highly significant ($P<0.001$) elevation of homovanillic acid, a metabolite of dopamine, but not of dopamine or salsolinol in the brains of rats given an ethanol challenge. Even more intriguing was the significant ($P<0.05$) elevation of striatal salsolinol following glucose administration. The same study revealed the presence of 1-carboxysalsolinol in the striata of rats and the caudate nucleus of human alcoholics with ethanol in the blood at autopsy. These results indicate that salsolinol in the brains of humans and animals could arise from the condensation of pyruvate, the end-product of glucose breakdown via glycolysis (see Light 1985), with dopamine to form 1-carboxysalsolinol. This, in turn, could then undergo decarboxylation to form salsolinol (Hirst *et al.* 1985; Sjöquist 1985). Energy metabolism thus appears to be of major importance in the formation of salsolinol independently of the presence of ethanol and its metabolites. Salsolinol is also present in many foods and in fermented beverages and dietary sources of this THIQ are also important sources which must be considered in any study of this nature (Smythe and Duncan 1985). And finally, Hirst *et al.* (1985) showed that ethanol dose, diet, gender, and social drinking level had major interactive effects on the appearance of salsolinol in the urine of human subjects.

The suggestion that the *in vivo* formation of mammalian THIQ-alkaloids, resulting from Pictet-Spengler condensation of biogenic amines and aldehydes, may play a major role in the genesis of alcoholism in man continues to be a controversial issue. In addition to the foregoing considerations, the lack of sufficiently specific or sensitive assay methodologies to detect these substances following ethanol administration continues to preclude definitive conclusions (Smythe and Duncan 1985). Although unproven, the hypothesis that THIQ's may play a significant role in physical dependency and addiction to alcohol remains very viable, at least in part (see Light 1986a for a discussion of the effects of alcohol on neural membrane systems and the role played by aldehyde adducts).

Multiple Metabolite Hypothesis and the Alcogene

Despite the foregoing caveats with respect to the *in vivo* production of biogenic amine-aldehyde adducts as the *direct* result of ethanol intake, abundant evidence now exists that aldehyde products are, in fact, formed in brain tissue following alcohol administration in rodents and humans. Whether these products are generated by altered redox balances, saturation of alcohol and aldehyde dehydrogenases by alcohol and acetaldehyde, condensation between ethanol-derived acetaldehyde and pyruvate deriving from glucose metabolism, or are absorbed directly from dietary sources or a combination of all of the above processes remains unclear.

Acetaldehyde, the immediate metabolite resulting from ethanol metabolism, is known to induce abnormally high levels of alcohol consumption by rats. Acetaldehyde is also known to be markedly increased in alcoholic human subjects over those in non-alcoholic controls following a given dose of ethanol (Lieber 1982). This is probably due to a combination of metabolic abnormalities (engorged and disrupted mitochondria and stimulation of microsomal enzymes, for example) and genetic factors (altered or unusual alcohol and aldehyde dehydrogenase activity). Elevated acetaldehyde levels, a shift in the redox state toward a reducing milieu (see Light 1985), and saturation of central alcohol dehydrogenase by exogenous ethanol could all contribute to a buildup of the intermediate aldehyde metabolites of catecholamines and indoleamines. The putative accumulation of these aminealdehydes and acetaldehyde are thought by many investigators to undergo the spontaneous Pictet-Spengler condensation described above to form THIQ's (salsolinol and tetrahydropapaveroline) and tetrahydro-β-carbolines. Salsolinol is known to be present in high levels in the dopamine-rich regions of the brain of alcoholic persons at autopsy, and β-carbolines have been reported in the brains of rats following ethanol administration (Myers 1985). All of these substances produce markedly increased voluntary alcohol intake by rats and mice as described above.

These considerations have led to the general conception of a *multiple metabolite* hypothesis concerning the biological factors which promote the genesis of alcoholism in human beings (Myers 1978, 1985). Most of the following material about this idea is abstracted from Myers (1985), who postulates that abnormally high levels of THIQ's and THBC's in the cerebrospinal fluid and/or brain tissue of alcoholic individuals may be caused by one or more defects in enzymatic reaction(s): "The intriguing possibility exists that the enzyme, aldehyde dehydrogenase . . ., in one or more of its isoenzyme forms, could be partially responsible for the formation of the adducts in brain tissue" (Myers 1985, p. 203).

As described above, both alcohol and aldehyde dehydrogenases, the enzymes by which the bulk of ingested alcohol is converted into acetate, are normally involved in the breakdown of the aminealdehydes produced by MAO and COMT acting upon the neurotransmitters dopamine, norepinephrine and serotonin (Figure 8). In the mammalian brain, the aldehydes of dopamine (DOPAL) and serotonin (SERAL) are usually predominantly oxidized to their corresponding acids, whereas the aldehydes of norepinephrine are primarily reduced to the corresponding alcohols (Tottmar 1985). In the absence of an exogenous alcohol load, the principal function of aldehyde dehydrogenase is directed toward the oxidation of DOPAL and SERAL (Figure 10A), and only trace amounts of acetaldehyde would be generated by the oxidation of the small amounts of endogenous ethanol produced by bacterial fermentation within the intestine.

When the system is challenged by an alcohol loading (Figure 10B), aldehyde dehydrogenase would be preferentially diverted for the metabolic breakdown of acetaldehyde, which is highly toxic. It is suggested (Myers 1985) that this could produce a transitory increase in the level of DOPAL, which could then undergo Pictet-Spengler condensation with its parent amine, dopamine, to form THPV (Figures 9B and 10B). Should the enzyme be more or less equally shared between the ethanol-derived and biogenic amine-derived aldehyde metabolites, acetaldehyde would tend to accumulate and presumably could then condense with dopamine to form salsolinol (Figures 9A and 10B). These aldehyde products are thought to exert their main effects upon certain opiate receptors in the brain, as discussed above. These THIQ's are hypothesized as providing a major neurochemical substrate for the biological "craving" of the alcohol-dependent individual for alcohol (Myers 1985). [An even more important mechanism underlying alcohol addiction appears to involve the response of neural membranes to the fluidizing effects of alcohol; a detailed account of this is given by Light 1986a.] According to Myers (1985, p. 211), "the unusually persistent effect of a TIQ in causing a permanent enhancement in alcohol consumption implies a conformational shift in receptor protein in the brain."

Tetrahydro-β-carbolines are as potent as THIQ's in producing

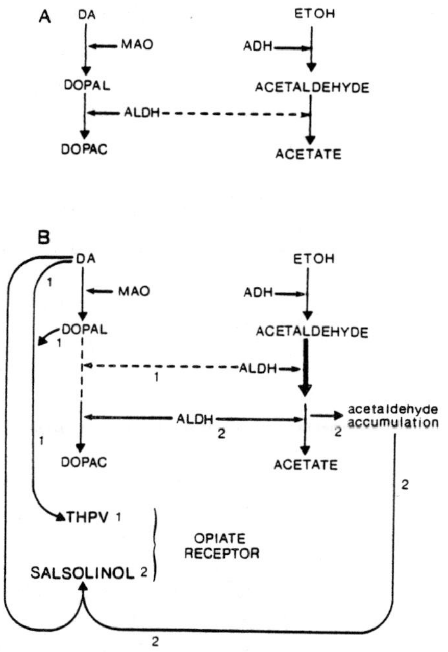

Figure 10. Neurotransmitter Catabolism and Ethanol. A. Normal metabolism of neurotransmitter (dopamine) and ethanol. Aldehyde dehydrogenase is involved in the oxidation of both the aminealdehyde metabolite (dopaldehyde) and the small amounts of circulating acetaldehyde resulting from the oxidation of ethanol deriving from fermentation by the intestinal bacteria. In the absence of a significant challenge of exogenous alcohol, the principal function of aldehyde dehydrogenase is directed toward the breakdown of neurotransmitters. **B.** Alcohol loading and THIQ formation. When the system is subjected to a significant ethanol challenge, aldehyde dehydrogenase would be diverted toward the oxidation of the highly toxic acetaldehyde into acetate. If the bulk of aldehyde dehydrogenase were preferentially occupied in detoxifying acetaldehyde (pathway 1), the conversion of dopaldehyde (DOPAL) would be inhibited, resulting in its increase and eventual condensation with its parent amine, dopamine (DA) to form THPV (see also Figure 9). In cases where aldehyde dehydrogenase is shared more or less equally by both the neurotransmitter and ethanol metabolic routes (pathway 2), more acetaldehyde would tend to accumulate than could be detoxified by the amount of available enzyme. This acetaldehydecould then condense with dopamine to form another THIQ, salsolinol. Both THPV and salsolinol could become sequestered in brain tissue and occupy opiate receptor sites, thereby mediating addictive alcohol consumption. DA = dopamine; MAO = monoamine oxidase; DOPAL = dopaldehyde; DOPAC = 3, 4-dihydroxyphenylacetic acid, the oxidation product of dopaldehyde; ETOH = ethanol; ADH = alcohol dehydrogenase; ALDH = aldehyde dehydrogenase; THPV = tetrahydropapaveroline. Based on several figures by Myers (1985).

elevated drinking behavior, yet they are also known to be powerful antagonists of certain benzodiazepine receptors in the central nervous system.[34] Myers (1985) suggests that the *in vivo* synthesis of THBC's resulting from alcohol metabolism could produce an anxiety state which might stimulate exaggerated alcohol consumption to relive the induced anxiety. This would presumably result in the generation of still more THBC's, producing in turn more drinking for symptomatic relief. Fear and anxiety would thus grow in an alcoholic individual over time.

Acetaldehyde has also been reported to condense with the endogenous opioids, methionine- and leucine-enkephalins to form Schiff's bases,

[34]The benzodiazepines or "minor tranquilizers" include such anti-anxiety drugs as Librium (chlordiazepoxide), Valium (diazepam), and Dalmane. The last is used primarily as a hypnotic for treating insomnia. Xanax (alprazolam) also belongs to this group of drugs and is used to treat anxiety and depression. In addition to their sedative-hypnotic and anti-anxiety properties, they are also used as anticonvulsants and as centrally-acting skeletal muscle relaxants. Although these drugs are among the safest, the therapeutic index being on the order of 100:1, tolerance and tachyphylaxis do develop, so that greater doses are soon needed to produce the desired effect. Continuous use of these drugs can result in a serious physical addiction and a dangerous withdrawal syndrome similar to that produced by barbiturates. Benzoadiazepines act upon specific receptors in the brain and spinal cord which are closely associated with GABA (gamma-aminobutyric acid) and glycine receptor complexes. [GABA is the most widely distributed inhibitory neurotransmitter in the brain; glycine fills that role in the spinal cord.] Ethanol and the barbiturates, in addition to their known membrane-fluidizing effects (see Light 1986a), also enhance the effects of GABA-benzodiazepine receptor complexes. Both GABA and the benzodiazepines activate specific receptors which open chloride ion channels. The influx of Cl^- hyperpolarizes the postsynaptic membrane, producing an inhibitory postsynaptic potential (see Light 1986a). The main site of action in the brain appears to be the limbic system, where these agents alleviate anxiety.

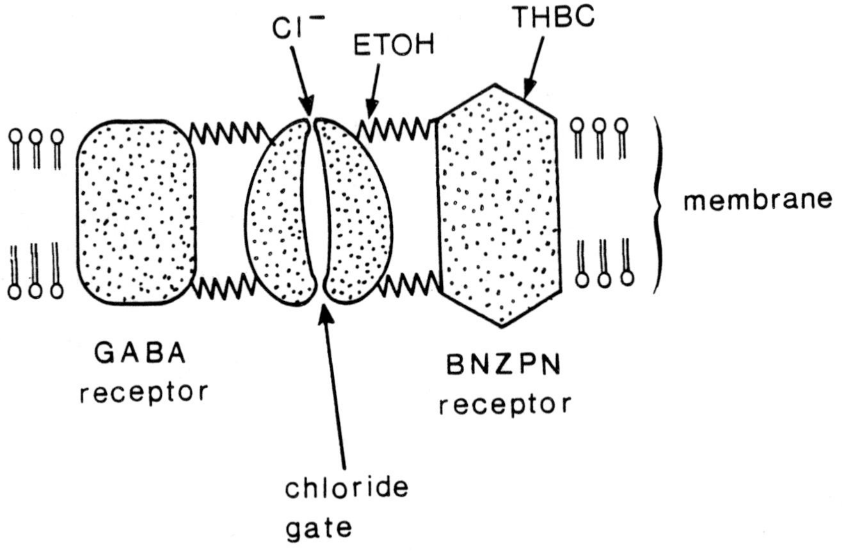

which then undergo ring closure to produce aldehyde adducts with negligible opiate activity (Summers 1985). Met-enkephalin is about 300 times more active than the corresponding aldehyde adduct in inhibiting contractions in mouse vas deferens, and about 100 times more potent in guinea pig assay. Leu-enkephalin is some 550 to 70 times more potent than its acetaldehyde adduct in the vas deferens and ileum assays, respectively. Such reactions between enkephalins and acetaldehyde to produce adducts with greatly reduced activity may also occur *in vivo* during ethanol intake. Such a reduction in endogenous opioid activity could be expected to produce an anxiety state similar to that described above for β-carbolines (see Light 1986a for a discussion of these compounds).

Thus, similar manifestations of abnormal alcohol consumption could develop even though THIQ's on the one hand and THBC's and enkephalin-aldehyde adducts on the other operate through different amine-aldehyde adduct-receptor mechanisms (Myers 1985). There is experimental support for this idea: when 1,2,3,4-tetrahydro-β-carboline is injected into rat hippocampus which contains both opiate and benzodiazepine receptors, an initial, extremely intense fear reaction is followed by abnormally high voluntary ethanol consumption in rats with an otherwise low preference for alcohol. Moreover, there appears to be a genetically predetermined susceptibility for this response to THBC administration. Several lines of rodents have been bred which tend to select or reject ethanol and water solutions; these lines are designated as being "addicted" or "non-addicted," respectively.

These considerations have given rise to the concept of an *alcogene* (Myers 1985). This notion is based upon the model of the *oncogene,* a gene encoding for a specific biological abnormalities under certain circumstances which predispose an individual to a given form of cancer.[35] Like oncogenes, the hypothesized alcogene would presumably be an integral part of the genetic complement in all cells, including neurons, in those individuals carrying the gene. Like oncogenes, alcogenes would produce no injury unless stimulated into activity by an enzyme such as

[35] Oncogenes are components of the genome of normal cells, and they typically encode for polypeptides essential to normal cellular function. The activity of cellular oncogenes can be unleashed or greatly intensified by a variety of carcinogens which act as transcriptional promoters (Figure 11) or deregulators, or by certain retroviruses which contain the viral RNA equivalent of the cellular oncogene. The cellular oncogene is grossly overexpressed, resulting in transformed cells run amok. Carcinogens and oncogene-bearing retroviruses turn "friend into foe," by directly stimulating excessive activity of the oncogene itself, or possibly by inhibiting one or more other genes that normally police the activity of the oncogene (Bishop 1982). The bottom line appears to be that transformed cells are simply overwhelmed with what are otherwise normal proteins engaged in normal cellular functions.

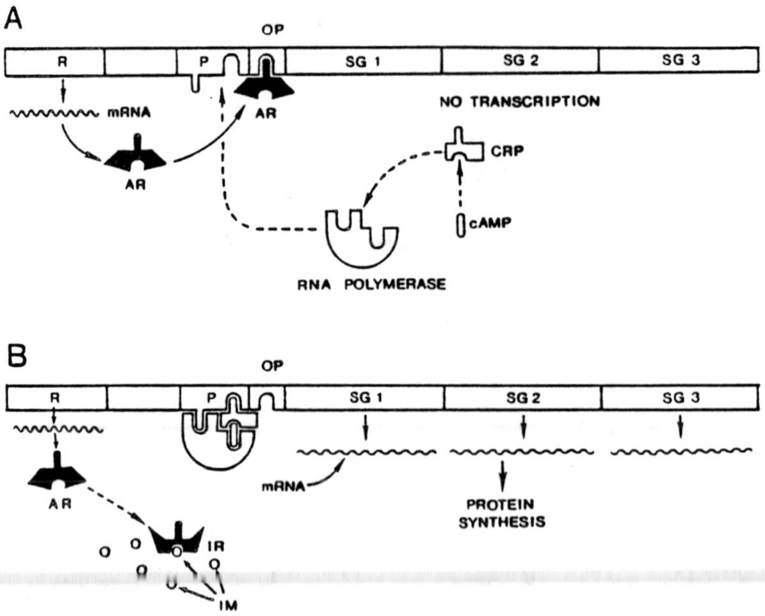

Figure 11. Induction of an Inducible Gene System. This model of an inducible gene system is based upon that involved in the production of β-galactosidase in the common intestinal bacterium of human beings, *Escherichia coli.* This enzyme begins the process of breaking down lactose, commonly known as "milk sugar," and is coded for by the *lac gene.* Two additional enzymes which are required for the further metabolism of lactose are located next to the lac gene; these three genes are labelled *structural genes* 1, 2, and 3 in the figure. A specific *repressor protein* is bound to the DNA at a site known as the *operator* when no *inducer molecules* (in this case, lactose itself) are present. Transcription is induced when RNA polymerase (see also Figure 2) is attached to the *promoter site* located next to the operator. In order for RNA polymerase to recognize the promoter gene, it must be combined with a *cyclic AMP receptor protein,* which in turn, must be combined with cyclic AMP. **A.** In an inducible gene system, active repressor protein is produced by the *regulator gene,* and under normal circumstances when no inducer molecules are present it attaches to the operator gene. Because of its size and shape, it overlaps part of the promoter, thus preventing the RNA polymerase complex from attaching and initiating transcription. **B.** When present, inducer molecules bind to the repressor protein, causing a configurational change so that the latter can no longer attach to the operator. The promoter is now uncovered and the RNA polymerase complex can attach to it and initiate transcription. All three structural genes are transcribed into one long mRNA molecule, which is then translated into all three lactose-metabolizing enzymes by the ribosomes. When the inducer molecule has been metabolically cleared from the body, the repressor protein changes back to its ground-state configuration and again occupies the operator, displacing RNA polymerase, and stopping transcription. Oncogenes are part of the normal genome of the individual, and normally cause no harm unless stimulated into activity (and probably overwhelming *hyperactivity*) by carcinogens. In a similar manner, alcohol or its metabolite acetaldehyde, might act as an inducing molecule which disinhibits the promoter of the hypothesized alcogene (see text), thus altering the normal functioning of the cell analogous to the way in which activated oncogenes produce cellular transformation, which can then eventually lead to cancer. R = regulator gene which codes for the repressor protein; P = promoter gene; OP = operator gene; SG 1-3 = the three structural genes of the operon coding for proteins which break down the inducer molecules (IM); AR = active repressor; cAMP = cyclic adenosine monophosphate; CRP = cAMP receptor protein; IR = inactivated repressor.

aldehyde dehydrogenase. Alcohol, acetaldehyde, or another metabolite could act as a promoter (see Figure 11), interacting with the alcogene to alter the normal function of the cell analogous to the way in which cellular transformation is produced by the activated oncogene.

As stated by Myers (1985, p. 214):

> That certain brain mechanisms potentially involved in the drinking of alcohol may co-vary with the genetic make-up of the organism is well-known. For example, the cerebral concentration of monoamines differ in rat strains exhibiting phenotypically divergent patterns of alcohol ingestion . . . Further, C57 and DBA mice show different levels of alcohol in [the] brain and acetaldehyde in [the] blood following an alcohol challenge . . . [and] selective destruction of catechole- and indoleamine pathways by neurotoxins . . . affects alcohol self-selection differentially in several strains of rats . . . Thus alcogenes may be coded for neurotransmitter activity in a discrete area of the brain, which varies according to strain . . . or to enzyme activity in [the] brain and liver . . .

It has also been suggested by several authors that alcoholism may be associated with other disorders known to be genetically inherited. When two or more genes are located fairly close together on the same arm of a chromosome, they tend to be inherited together. [The reader is referred to Appendix I for a discussion of the mechanics of genetic segregation and inheritance patterns.] The closer two genes are, moreover, the less likely they are to be separated by translocations and other chromosome mutation events. If such a linkage between alcoholism and other genetic traits could be established, the other trait[s] could then serve as genetic *markers* to establish the likelihood of alcoholism in a given individual.

Colorblindness is one such potential marker proposed by several Chilean investigators (Cruz-Coke and Varela 1966; 1970). These workers noted a very close association between alcoholism and colorblindness, and because the gene for colorblindness is known to lie on the X-chromosome, they postulated a recessive sex-linked model for the inheritance of alcoholism. Because of its recessive nature, the allele for alcoholism would readily be expressed in the hemizygous or male (XY) condition, but only rarely in females (XX) in the uncommon event that two recessive alleles were to come together in the same individual. This model would seem on the face of it to explain why alcoholism is so much more common in males than females. Later studies showed, however, that the colorblindness associated with alcoholism in this population is reversible after a few weeks of abstinence. The "marker," then, is not genetically linked with alcoholism at all, but is the consequence of alcohol toxicity perhaps involving liver disease or some other metabolic complication such as interference with retinol-retinal interactions (see Light 1986a). Moreover, this model cannot account for the fact that alcoholism seems to be strongly inherited by males from their fathers, and *not* from their mothers. Since fathers can only pass on Y-chromosomes to their sons, an X-linked transmission cannot possibly account for the observed patterns of male inheritance of alcoholism.

Electroencephalogram characteristics taken under standard conditions (relaxed with eyes closed) and in the absence of disturbing influences such as fatigue, brain disease or severe metabolic disorder appear to be genetically determined (Vogel and Motulsky 1979). This is particularly true in the case of the resting α-rhythm; twin and family studies indicate that this trait is under simple dominant inheritance. EEG α-wave activity appears to be formed by complex neurophysiological processes originating in the cerebral cortex which are modulated by thalamic "pacemakers" which are in turn influenced by the reticular activating system (see Light 1986a). High R.A.S. activity maintains arousal and results in a poorly developed and desynchronized α-rhythm.

Individuals with well developed and stable resting α-rhythms indicative of personality stability and lack of neurosis show little change in α-activity following an ethanol challenge. In contrast, those with poorly developed and desynchronized α-rhythms characteristic of high tonic arousal exhibit a strong response to ethanol in which their α-waves become stronger, stable and synchronized (Figure 12). In other words, these tense and anxious people become relaxed and more mellow following alcohol intake and this is reflected in a stabilized and prominent α-rhythm. Normally relaxed and non-tense individuals do not respond nearly as strongly to alcohol. These responses are highly concordant in monozygotic twins but not so in dizygotic twins (in some cases the latter are even discordant). This alteration in EEG activity is not associated with blood alcohol content and it persists long after most of the alcohol has been cleared from the body. It has been suggested (Vogel and Motulsky 1979) that alcohol acts to modulate a desynchronizing input from the reticular formation in those tense individuals with a strong positive EEG response to ethanol. This, in turn, improves the synchronizing function of the pacemaker centers in the thalamus. The normally strong pacemaker function in the thalami of normal controls is not subject to reticular influence to the same extent and the response to alcohol is relatively small.

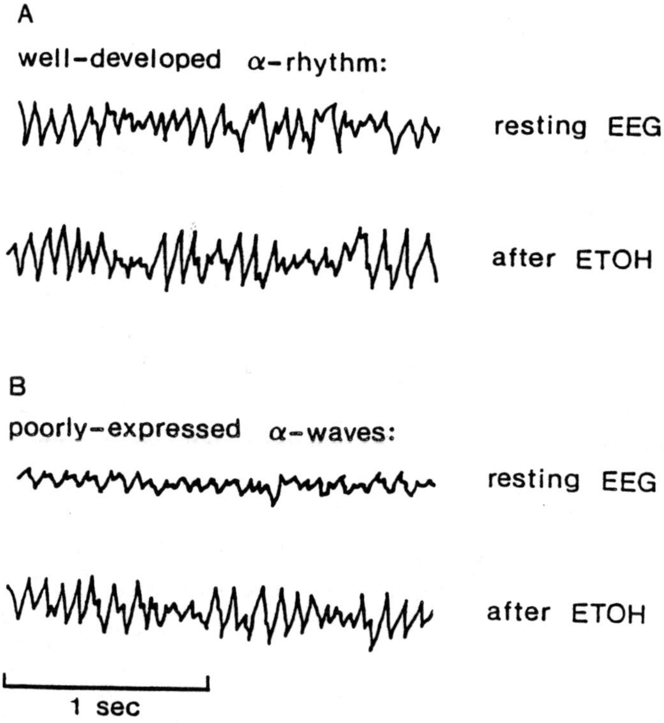

Figure 12. Effect of Alcohol Upon Normal and Abnormal α-Rhythms. A. Well-developed resting occipital α-rhythm before and after an alcohol challenge. Relatively little effect on the α-pattern is produced by alcohol. **B.** Poorly expressed α-waves associated with a high state of arousal and anxiety. Note the dramatic change produced by alcohol; the resulting strong and synchronized α-pattern is associated with a subjective feeling of relief and well-being in such subjects. Based upon figures by Vogel and Motulsky (1979).

A similarly poorly developed and destabilized α-rhythm is also seen among alcoholics, which specifically resembles that seen in twins showing the strong alcohol response just described. Recent evidence (Pollock *et al.* 1983; Curran 1983) indicates that the biological sons of alcoholic fathers also exhibit such poorly developed and desynchronized α-patterns *prior to having ever been exposed to alcohol.*[36] Furthermore, these α-waves likewise smooth out and become significantly stronger in response to an alcohol challenge. None of the age-matched controls (sons of non-alcoholic fathers) exhibited any of these abnormal responses. These aberrant brainwave patterns in abstinent chronic alcoholics were previously assumed to result from alcohol-induced brain damage, but the fact that they exist in the sons of alcoholics prior to any ethanol insult

[36]Nor had the mothers drunk alcohol during pregnancy, which rules out any possible effects of alcohol on the developing fetal brain.

strongly suggests that they are genetically predetermined. Prealcoholic, poorly developed α-waves are known to be associated with stress, anxiety and dysphoria; the EEG's of such individuals respond to ethanol by much greater decreases in fast α-activity and increases in slow α-activity relative to normal controls. This appears to reflect the increased psychic tension and exaggerated relief obtained from alcohol intake seen in alcoholics. As stated by Curran (1983) and quoted in Light (1986a, page 85): "For those with a genetic predisposition to alcoholism, alcohol may have a positive reinforcing effect by slowing brain activity. Thirty-nine percent of the biological sons of alcoholic fathers showed these aberrant brain waves, which were generated primarily in the hippocampus and limbic system. This figure closely approximates the reports of other investigators that 30 to 40 percent of the sons of alcoholic fathers will themselves also become alcoholic." [See also below.]

Similarly, Vogel and Motulsky (1979, page 517) observed that ". . . genetic susceptibility [to high tonic arousal and dysphoria] may lead to different phenotypic effects, depending on the sociocultural conditions of the environment. In a western society with its strong emphasis on social drinking, the genetically susceptible individual is endangered to become an alcoholic. In a Buddhist setting, the same person would probably become one especially dedicated to meditation."[37]

Evoked potentials (EP's) are abrupt changes in electrical activity in the brain produced by sensory stimuli such as patterns of light, geometric or random figures, tones, and the like. They reflect the net electrical activity in the population of neurons in the region where the electrode is implanted or attached which are affected by the stimulus. Unlike the spontaneous, background electrophysiological activity of the EEG, evoked potentials are elicited in response to a visual or auditory stimulus. The neuroelectrical activity of the EP is also time-locked to the signal and is elicited each time the stimulus is presented. In contrast, the background EEG "noise" in which it is embedded is not time-locked to the signal. Thus, although EP's are generally too small to be distinguished from the large, background changes in voltage of the EEG, by repeating the stimulus many times and feeding the results through an *averaging computer,* the evoked response emerges clearly from the background EEG noise. For a given individual, averaged EP's to a specific

[37] Alpha-activity can also be enhanced by meditation and biofeedback techniques, and this is associated with a subjective sense of well-being and tranquility. These activities also appear to involve elevated enkephalin activity, which similarly promotes subjective feelings of well-being (see Light 1986a for further discussion).

signal are quite stable over time, all other things being equal. Although a given stimulus produces similar EP patterns in different subjects, *distinct individual differences are also evident*! Furthermore, EP's also vary with the internal state of the subject—for example, the state of alertness, degree of expectation, or familiarity of the subject with the signal. And finally, the waveforms of evoked potentials reflect how the subject interprets the signal—that is, its significance or meaning, as well as any decision-making process that may be involved.

Averaged evoked potentials recorded in response to a repeated stimulus produce a characteristic positive-negative-positive [P1-N1-P2] waveform occurring between 60 and 250 milliseconds following the signal (Figure 13). These waveforms are generally differentiated into two major component sets as follows:

(1) *Early Component:* occurs <100 msec after the signal [P1-N1]; this component is mainly related to the physical characteristics of the stimulus, for example, the intensity or wave frequency of a light or sound stimulus.

(2) *Late Components:* occurs >100 msec after the signal [N1-P2]; mainly reflects psychological and associative processes, for example, habituation and selection of relevant (target) and irrelevant (non-target) stimuli [see below].

The P1-N1-P2 waveform is elicited in response to the passive reception of a stimulus by the subject. More sophisticated studies involve the recording and evaluation of *event-related potentials* (ERP's) which require the subject to actively undertake specific tasks while the ERP is being recorded. For example, target selection tasks involve the detection of a rarely occurring target stimulus intermingled in a series of often occurring non-target signals. Event-related potentials produced in response to frequently presented non-target stimuli elicit only N1-P2 late components. Rarely presented target signals, on the other hand, elicit N1-P2 as well as P3 components. The P3 component consists of a large positive potential occurring between 300 and 500 milliseconds after presentation of the target signal, and which involves discrimination of the target from non-target signals. Under normal circumstances, the greater the deviation of the rare target signal is from the non-target background noise, the more easily it can be discriminated and the larger the P3 amplitude will be (Figure 13).

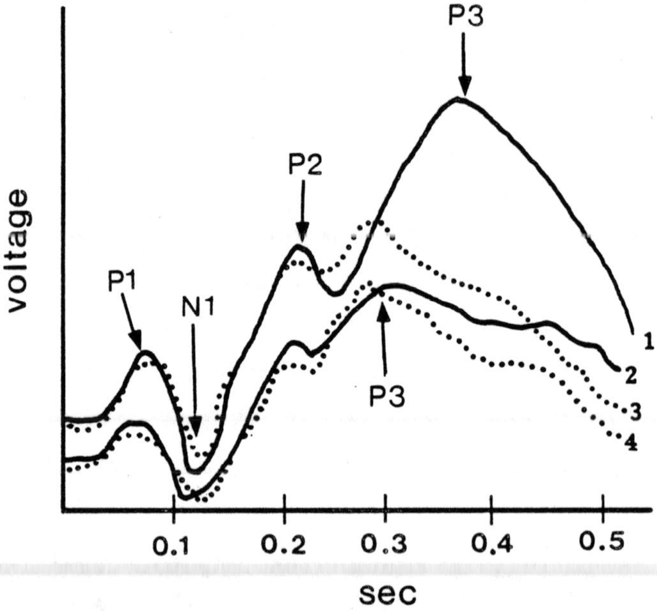

Figure 13. Evoked Potential Waveforms in Alcoholics and Non-alcoholics. Averaged evoked potentials to repetitive signals of any modality produce a characteristic positive-negative-positive [P1-N1-P2; = P100-N140-P200] waveform which occurs some 60-250 milliseconds after the stimulus is presented. This waveform is divided into early components occurring less than 100 msec, and late components occurring more than 100 msec following the stimulus. Early components reflect mainly the physical characteristics of the stimulus itself, such as intensity, and they are relatively resistant to the effects of alcohol. The late components reflect primarily psychological processes, such as habituation, and the association areas of the brain. The late components are very susceptible to alcohol-induced modification. If one or more target stimuli which must be differentiated by the subject from the background noise are added, producing event-related potentials (ERP's) a P3 [= P300] positive peak is obtained which occurs between 300 and 500 msec after the stimulus is applied. In the above figure, the solid lines represent the ERP response to a series of stimuli which include a target which must be discriminated from the background; the dotted lines represent signals not including a target signal. Curves 1 and 3 are those of non-alcoholic controls. The P1-N1 amplitudes are well developed, the P2 peak is very pronounced, and the P3 peak shows a much more dramatic response to target as contrasted with non-target stimuli. Curves 2 and 4 show the response of alcoholics to signals with and without a target. Note that the P1-N1-P2 amplitudes are much weaker than those of controls, and that the P3 peak is both highly reduced relative to control subjects, and that there is little difference between the response by alcoholics to target and non-target signals. These features suggest that there may be an underlying sensory filtering deficit in alcoholics. Based on several figures by Begleiter *et al.* (1984) and by Porjesz *et al.* (1985).

In a major review article, Porjesz and Begleiter (1985) discussed their own and others' work concerning the relationship of evoked potentials and event-related potentials to alcoholism. Much of the following is abstracted from that paper, although other appropriate literature is also cited.

Several studies have shown that alcohol administration results in a significant depression of late ERP components [N1-P2], whereas the early components are relatively resistant to such changes. The decrease in N1-P2 amplitudes produced by acute doses of ethanol is directly correlated to blood alcohol level, suggesting that alcohol exerts far greater inhibition over higher cognitive association areas than primary stimulus receiving areas of the brain. Non-alcoholic, healthy individuals exhibit an enhanced N1 response to relevant, target stimuli, whereas this component is reduced when presented with irrelevant signals.

Alcoholics have been consistently shown to exhibit evoked potentials with markedly reduced late component [N1-P2], but not early component [P1-N1] amplitudes (Beck *et al.* 1978; Dustman *et al.* 1979; Porjesz and Begleiter 1985). Furthermore, ERP studies using a variety of target-selection paradigms have revealed major decreases in late component [N1-P2 and P3] amplitudes, as well as delayed late component latencies reflecting reduced excitability. Abstinent alcoholics thus appear to manifest EP and ERP signatures which are very similar to those of normal persons under the influence of alcohol. Moreover, whereas normal people respond to relevant and irrelevant stimuli with enhanced and reduced N1 amplitudes, respectively, alcoholics exhibit the same low N1 amplitude regardless of the degree of signal relevance. This may reflect an underlying sensory filtering deficit in chronic alcoholics (Porjesz and Begleiter 1985).

In a separate study of the P3 component in a target-selection visual paradigm, Porjesz and colleagues (1980) recorded ERP's to targets (rarely occurring geometric shapes), non-targets (frequently occurring non-relevant shapes) and novel stimuli (rarely occurring, irrelevant, random shapes). All stimuli would be expected to elicit large N1 amplitudes, but only the rare signals should elicit P3 components. Alcoholics manifested a significantly depressed N1-P2 amplitude to all stimuli (target, non-target and novel signals) to levels consistent with an irrelevant stimulus modality—once again suggesting impaired sensory filtering processes in chronic alcoholics. And the late component P3 am-

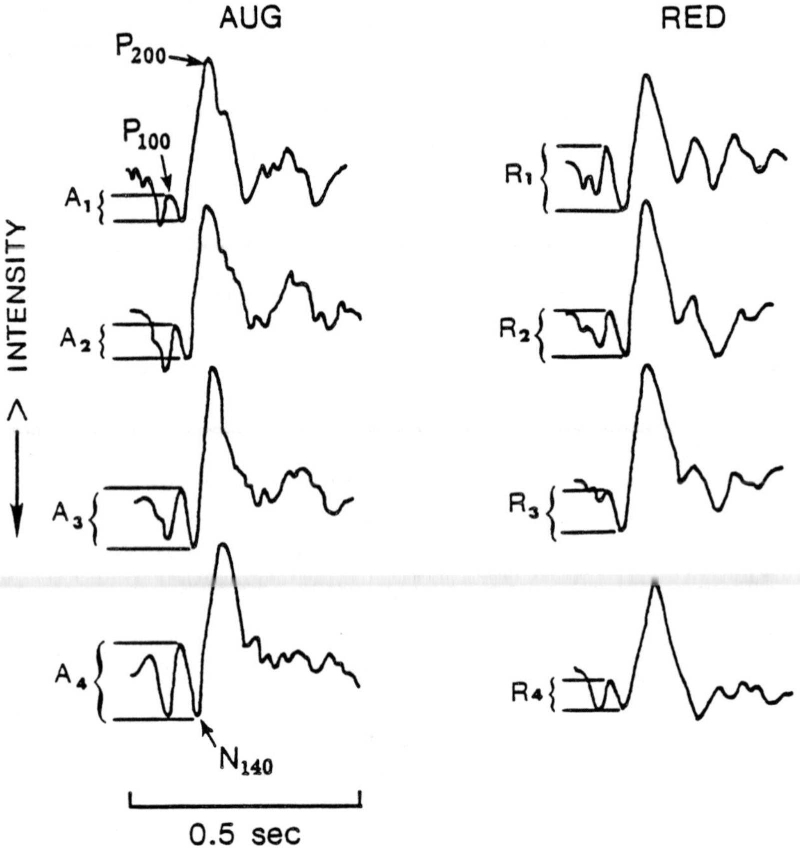

Figure 14. Visual Evoked Potentials in Augmenters and Reducers. Averaged evoked potentials to four increasing intensities of light flashes from top to bottom. The left series of EP's are those of an augmenter, exhibiting increasing P100-N140 amplitudes in response to increasing stimulus intensity. These increasing amplitudes are labelled A_1 through A_4. The right series of EP's are those of a reducer. Note that the P100-N140 amplitudes *decrease* in response to the increasing stimulus intensity. Augmenters given an ethanol challenge respond to a stimulus of increasing intensity by sharply reducing their augmentation. Several studies have shown that alcoholics tend to be strong augmenters who respond to alcohol by sharply decreasing their evoked P100-N140 amplitude. Both augmenters and alcoholics appear to suffer a significant sensory filtering deficit, and for alcoholics, at least, alcohol intake is associated with a welcome reduction in sensory stimulus bombardment.

plitudes were also markedly depressed or entirely absent in the alcoholic subjects in response to rare target signals which should have produced large P3 amplitudes. Unlike control subjects which exhibited differentially enhanced P3 amplitudes to target signals, alcoholics responded with identical low amplitude P3 waves (Figure 13) regardless of whether the signal being presented was a target or non-target—once again demonstrating an inability to distinguish between relevant and non-relevant stimuli, and suggesting an underlying brain dysfunction which impairs sensory filtering mechanisms (Porjesz and Begleiter 1985).

Studies on central nervous system excitability (Petrie 1978) have revealed two main types of responder profiles to stimulation:

(1) *Augmenters:* These individuals tend to exhibit amplified evoked potential responses to visual, auditory, or pain stimuli. Specifically, they respond to signals of increasing intensity (for example, flashes of light) with corresponding increases in the amplitudes of component P1[P100]-N1[N140][38] waveforms (Figure 14). Augmenters suffer relatively greater subjective pain when confronted with given intensities of painful stimuli, and they tend to consistently overestimate the size of visually presented objects such as blocks.

(2) *Reducers:* These persons tend to exhibit diminished evoked potential responses to stimuli of given intensities, and they show decreasing P100-N140 amplitudes in response to increasing stimulus intensity (Figure 14). Such individuals appear to be generally understimulated and they regularly underestimate the size of visually presented blocks. They exhibit a significantly greater tolerance for pain than do augmenters.[39]

Augmenters appear to be individuals who generally experience an excessive amount of sensory bombardment. These persons tend to try to avoid sensory overload by retreating into quiet and relatively inactive, solitary pursuits. They are more socially inhibited and they tend to have only a few intimate friends. Reducers, on the other hand, tend to experience sensory starvation for which they attempt to compensate by active participation in a variety of intense activities and undertakings. They appear to have many more friends than augmenters and more active social lives.

In addition to extreme augmenters and reducers, two other types of responders have been described: (a) *moderates,* who do not tend to greatly overestimate or underestimate the size of visually presented objects, and (b) *stimulus-governed* individuals, who tend to underestimate the dimen-

[38]The P1 component [= P100] is so-named because it occurs about 100 milliseconds after presentation of the stimulus; similarly, the N1 component [= N140] occurs about 140 milliseconds after the signal. The P2 [= P200] and P3 [= P300] late components are registered about 200 and between 300 and 500 milliseconds, respectively.

[39]This does not necessarily mean that reducers have a higher *pain threshold,* but rather that they experience a *reduction in perceived pain stimuli!* The total time a subject can endure a stream of sensory bombardment may be more important in tolerance for pain than is the pain threshold itself (Petrie 1978).

sions of large, visually presented objects by 6 mm or more, and to overestimate the size of small objects, again by more than 6 mm. The stimulus-governed response appears to be common among patients with various organic brain pathologies and in juvenile delinquents (Petrie 1978).

Alcohol is known to increase both perceptual reduction and tolerance for pain, and this effect is most pronounced among perceptual augmenters. As stated by Petrie (1978, pages 40-41):

> . . . if we break down our population into augmenters, moderates, and reducers, we find that after the consumption of alcohol it is the augmenters in whom the maximum and dramatic change is found, for they cease enlarging and begin to reduce. Diminished augmentation occurred in every one of the augmenters [studied by us, and] . . . the average change . . . [in this] group . . . had a P-value of .001. The moderates, however, showed almost no change at all. The reducers changed a little, though not so much as the augmenters; the direction of the change was to make them reduce slightly less . . .
>
> What all this means is that the consumption of as little as two ounces of alcohol is followed by a most significant increase in reduction in augmenters.

And again on page 43, Petrie notes that, "Not only does the reduction influence perceived size, weight, and pain, but the loudness of a sound of constant intensity is likely to be lessened after taking alcohol."

Both alcoholic and non-alcoholic augmenters respond to alcohol by exhibiting a marked decrease in augmentation. This is very similar to the exaggerated effect that alcohol exerts in alcoholics and about 40 percent of their biological offspring, in which poorly developed and chaotic resting α-rhythms (see above) become stronger, more stabilized and synchronized with alcohol intake (Figure 12). It is especially significant, then, that stimulus-response and evoked potential studies have consistently shown that alcoholics tend to be strong augmenters (Petrie 1978; Buchsbaum 1978; Porjesz and Begleiter 1985). Numerous investigators have observed that alcoholics appear to depend upon alcohol to inhibit their sensory input, and that alcoholics under the influence of high doses of alcohol show P100-N140 amplitude gradients much like those of sober controls. Alcohol appears to have a normalizing effect on several different CNS functions in alcoholic subjects, reducing tension (as manifested by converting abnormal α-waves into strong, normal-appearing patterns) and countering CNS hyperexcitability (as reflected by reducing EP augmentation) thought to derive from a deficit in cortical inhibition in alcoholics (Porjesz and Begleiter 1985).

As is true of EEG patterns (see above), evoked potential waveforms are under strong genetic determination (Buchsbaum 1978). Monozygotic (MZ) twins exhibit EP waveforms that are as concordant with each other as are EP's obtained from the same individual tested twice (Begleiter *et al.* 1984; Porjesz and Begleiter 1985). Buchsbaum (1974) found significantly higher intraclass correlation coefficients in monozygotic than in dizygotic twin pairs for three separate measurements of the P100 amplitude-intensity slope: the P100-N140 peak-to-trough amplitude, the 76-112 msec mean deviation measure, and the amplitude for a single coordinate of exactly 100 msec. For the MZ twin pairs, ranged from .54 to .68, whereas DZ intraclass correlations were near zero.[40] When the MZ correlation is more than twice the DZ correlation, simple additive genetic variance cannot account for the heritability, and several allelic loci and/or dominance, epistasis [suppression of the penetrance of a

[40]A composite population with a mean, μ, and a common variance, σ^2, [see footnote 28] will have a total variance, σ_T^2, consisting of two components: (1) σ^2, a measure of the variability of the X_{ij} measurements within each subpopulation, and (2) $\sigma_{\mu_i}^2$, a measure of the variation of the subpopulation means. Each of these components of the total variance, σ_T^2, are independent of each other. It can be shown that $\sigma_T^2 = \sigma_{\mu_i}^2 + \sigma^2$ for the composite population, and this parameter can be estimated for a sample by $s_T^2 = s^2 + s_{\mu_i}^2$. The intraclass correlation coefficient, ρ_i, can be estimated for a sample by:

$$r_i = \frac{s_{\mu_i}^2}{s_T^2} = \frac{s_{\mu_i}^2}{s^2 + s_{\mu_i}^2}$$

Intraclass correlation coefficients for MZ and DZ twins can be used to determine the relative importance of genetic and environmental factors involved in the phenotypic expression of a trait. The heritability value is given by:

$$h^2 = \frac{r_{i_{MZ}} - r_{i_{DZ}}}{1 - r_{i_{DZ}}};$$

this is also known as the H [Holzinger] index. As $r_{i_{MZ}}$ approaches 1, H also tends toward 1; when H = 1, the phenotypic variability is entirely determined by heredity. When $r_{i_{MZ}}$ tends toward 0, H likewise tends toward 0, and the phenotypic variation is due more to environmental factors. The phenotypic intrapair correlation coefficient is given by:

$$r_{P,\text{twins}} = \frac{V_P^B}{V_P^B + V_P^W},$$

where V_P^B = the phenotypic variance between pairs and V_P^W = the phenotypic variance within pairs (Vogel and Motulsky 1979). [Note that this is merely a variation of the equation for the intraclass correlation coefficient, r_i, given above.] Assumptions inherent in this model are (1) that MZ twins have the same genotype, (2) that DZ twins have differing genotypes, and (3) that both members of each twin pair are exposed to the same environment from conception onwards. The first two assumptions are valid, but the third may not always be so. In addition, the covariance between heredity and environment and the variance due to the interaction between genetic and environmental factors are assumed to be zero, and this is probably rarely the case (Vogel and Motulsky 1979).

gene by a nonallelic gene], or dominance interactions are likely to be involved (Buchsbaum 1978).

Begleiter and his colleagues (1984) recently reported that a group of biological sons of alcoholic fathers between the ages of 7 and 13 who had no previous exposure to alcohol exhibited the same reduced P3 [= P300] amplitudes in response to a stimulus seen in the alcoholics themselves. Since boys whose mothers were alcoholic were excluded from the study, any potential complicating factors arising from fetal alcohol effects were effectively eliminated. Because reaction times did not differ between the high-risk boys (biological sons of alcoholic fathers) and the low-risk controls (boys without an alcoholic parent), the marked differences in P300 amplitude (see Figure 13) are unlikely to be due to attentional differences. The observed P300 deficits in the high-risk group was even more striking for a difficult task than for a relatively easy one. This same phenomenon was also reported for abstinent alcoholics (see above) and it appears to reflect an underlying sensory filtering deficit.

Certain electrophysiological abnormalities in abstinent alcoholics, such as delayed brainstem potentials evoked in response to stimuli, improve considerably or remit entirely with increasing duration of abstinence from alcohol (Begleiter *et al.* 1984; Porjesz and Begleiter 1985). Others, however, especially evoked P300 waveforms remain abnormal even following several years of continuous sobriety. These investigators suggested that rather than being the result of years of heavy drinking, these P300 amplitude decrements probably antedate alcohol abuse. At least 36 percent of the sons of alcoholics were found to manifest some ERP abnormality prior to any exposure to alcohol. This figure is in good agreement with the proportion of the sons of alcoholics manifesting abnormal EEG's which are dramatically improved with alcohol intake, and the percentage of the sons of alcoholics who eventually become alcoholic themselves (see discussions above).

An intriguing idea was recently proposed relative to genetic susceptibility to alcoholism and the length of time an ethnic or cultural group has been exposed to alcohol (Milam and Ketchum 1981). These authors suggest that Jews and Italians have had access to large quantities of alcohol for more than 7,000 years, and their rates for alcoholism tend to be low. The rest of Europe including Scandinavia, he states, became exposed to significant quantities of alcohol about 1,500 years ago. This is said to correlate with the relatively higher rates of alcoholism found in those countries. And Native American peoples who exhibit extreme rates of severe alcoholism did not become exposed to large amounts of alcohol until about 300 years ago. Milam and Ketchum propose that natural selection—those evoluntionary forces that tend to weed out those less fit individuals over milennia—would gradually eliminate those individuals who are genetically susceptible to alcoholism. And this selective process would become more advanced as time progresses. Therefore, they argue, those cultures with the longest exposures to alcohol would show the greatest genetic resistance to developing alcoholism simply because most of the genes predisposing to that disease would have been eliminated.

There are several difficulties with this interesting idea. In order for genes to be selectively eliminated from a population, selection must operate *before reproduction occurs*. The individuals carrying these deleterious genes must be eliminated from the reproductive pool either by early death or by being outcompeted for mating partners in one way or another. An individual who is sexually unattractive or deformed or who is unable to acquire territory or effectively challenge rivals, for example, very likely would be unable to obtain a mate and reproduce. There is no evidence that alcoholics are unable to acquire mating partners and to produce children relative to anyone else in human society. Alcoholism typically works its ravages upon the alcoholic person in later life *after* he or she has reproduced. Furthermore, alcoholics are prone to sexual and other acting-out behavior and the likelihood is that they are *more likely* to reproduce both within and outside of marriage. Probably the majority of unwanted babies who are put up for adoption in western society are the progeny of alcoholics. It is probably true enough, I grant, that children who are abused and battered to death by their parents are mostly found in alcoholic families. But I doubt that this makes a significant decrement in the overall number produced.

In the case of Jewish society with its emphasis upon intellectual abilities (Jews typically run 10 to 15 IQ points higher than the general white population) and its abhorrence of drunkenness, it is indeed possible that such a selection might occur. I can imagine that Jewish women would be reluctant to marry anyone whose parents were alcoholic, especially in the past when marriages were largely arranged by the couples' parents and family. It is possible that such a selection as Milam and Ketchum hypothesize could have worked to reduce the rates of alcoholism among Jews. But such a trend, if it did exist, appears to be crumbling in today's society. I know a great many Jewish women who married non-Jewish alcoholics, and there are significant numbers of them in Al-Anon today. Jewish women not infrequently exhibit enabling behaviors and a need to play a suffering and martyrlike role in order to act out feelings of guilt. Such women flock to alcoholics like ducks to water. The children of such marriages will exhibit high rates of alcoholism. The rate at which Jews in general are marrying non-Jews has many Jewish leaders worried that they will be assimilated out of existence by the rest of society.

There is another facet of alcoholism that is rarely examined. Like most things, alcoholism has some positive aspects as well. Alcoholics as a group tend to exhibit many of society's finest attributes. They are extraordinarily talented and creative and, prior to the onset of alcoholic deterioration, they are among society's hardest driving, most ambitious, and accomplished individuals. They very commonly rise to the top of their professions. They make a significant proportion of mankind's major accomplishments and they rule nations and win major military engagements. And they have done this throughout all of human history. Society *needs* its alcoholics! The allies would never have won World War II had not Sir Winston Churchill, an alcoholic, been who he was and where he was at the time. And I doubt whether the Union forces would have won our own Civil War without the brilliant generalship of Ulysses S. Grant, also an alcoholic. I don't mean to suggest that one has to be an alcoholic in order to be a brilliant general—Douglas MacArthur and Dwight Eisenhower are eloquent testimony to that. What I *am* saying is that a huge number of society's greatest contributors in politics, the military, the arts and the sciences *are* alcoholics, and without them the world would be a drearier place indeed. I cannot imagine a world without the works of Ernest Hemingway or F. Scott Fitzgerald or the screen performances of W.C. Fields, Marilyn Monroe, Judy Garland or even, it seems, William Holden, to name but a tiny few.

Alcoholism is a terrible tragedy to those afflicted with it and their families. But it is a two-edged sword. Most of society's violent crimes, homicides, suicides and certainly traffic fatalities are committed by alcohol abusers. But a great deal of our most cherished treasures we also owe to our alcoholics. They give every bit as much, if not even more, than they take away or destroy.

My own feeling is that alcoholism is by and large a selectively neutral phenotype and that, with the possible exception of traditional Jewish society, it persists in the population according to Hardy-Weinberg equilibrium (see Appendix 1). As devastating an illness as it is, it does not for the most part incapacitate its victims until late adulthood, long after they have left progeny to carry on their genetic inheritance. And alcoholics are as successful, if not more so, than any other group. They occupy all socioeconomic levels and they often wield great power. On an evolutionary basis, there seems to be nothing maladaptive about alcoholism as a phenotype.

FETAL ALCOHOL SYNDROME

THAT ALCOHOL consumption by pregnant women can result in deformed and retarded offspring has been known and commented upon since early Biblical times (*Judges* 13:7) and somewhat later by Aristotle, and very occasionally during the 19th and early part of the 20th centuries (see Streissguth *et al.* 1980). The term *fetal alcohol syndrome* was coined in 1973 by Drs. K.L. Jones and D.W. Smith (1973) for those offspring of chronically alcoholic women exhibiting a characteristic cluster of similar facial abnormalities, mental and physical retardation, and psychomotor disturbances. This particular combination of effects appears to occur only among the offspring of chronic and severely alcoholic women and the manifestation of the fetal alcohol syndrome constellation is in itself sufficient to warrant the diagnosis of maternal alcoholism (Streissguth *et al.* 1980). Fetal alcohol syndrome has been clearly demonstrated in animal models (mice) as the direct result of *two small challenges of ethanol* to pregnant dams, including the characteristic facial features typical of human cases (Sulik *et al.* 1981), about which more below. In recent years the number of reports of this syndrome has increased enormously and literally hundreds of cases have been described from several countries in Europe, North America, South Africa and Australia.

Despite the overwhelming and unequivocal evidence that the drinking of alcohol can and does cause congenital deformities and retardation—even in moderate or small amounts—our cultural imperative that drinking is not only appropriate and even "good" for you, and the almost automatic conclusion that *not* drinking is therefore "bad," continues to fuel an often acrimonious debate about whether pregnant women should be advised not to drink (there appears to be no such controversy with regard to other drugs) during the terms of their pregnancies (see, for example, Kolata 1981). That so many professional "authorities" persist in allowing their own hidden agenda about the subject to override common sense and the overwhelming burden of the evidence is a glaring reflection of the ambivalence with which we as a society regard beverage alcohol.[41]

The full fetal alcohol syndrome (FAS) has been consistently described by a number of authors as including the following features (for example, Rosett 1979; Chernoff 1980; Streissguth *et al.* 1980; Sulik *et al.* 1981):

(1) Growth deficiency in weight and length at birth which persists so that postnatal catch-up does not generally occur; FAS children are typically under the third percentile[42] in height, weight, and head circumference. These children have reduced adipose reserves at birth and this reduction becomes more pronounced postnatally and they are often extremely thin.

(2) A variety of central nervous system deficits, including mild to moderate mental retardation, with a mean of about 68 (mildly retarded) but with a wide range in scores (16 to 106 in the United States—Streissguth *et al.* 1980); as is evident from the I.Q. range, a few FAS children have normal intelligence, but most are significantly handicapped. Associated CNS features include small head size or *microcephaly,* poor coordination, irritability, hyperactive behavior and poor attention spans.

(3) A characteristic suite of facial features that in themselves are diagnostic for FAS (see Figure 15):

(a) short *palpebral fissures* or eye slits, often associated with small, myopic eyes, *ptosis* or drooping of the upper eyelid (typically associated with paralysis of the *oculomotor* or third cranial nerve or of sympathetic innervation), and *strabismus* or squinting and deviation of the axes of the eyes such as occurs in "cross-eye"; an *epicanthic fold* or "almond-eye" such as seen in Oriental persons is commonly present.[43]

---

[41] This same basic lack of proportion is seen in the continuing insistence in certain professional quarters that alcoholics not only can but *should* be reprogrammed to drink "socially." Quite aside from the ideological (one hesitates to use the word "theoretical" in this context) convictions these authors may entertain about the cause(s) of alcoholism, the gross medical consequences alone of chronic alcohol abuse mandate the immediate complete, and *permanent* cessation of alcohol intake by alcoholic patients. To counsel otherwise is sheer quackery! One does not attempt to make a "social smoker" out of an emphysema patient by way of analogy.

[42] Two-thirds of all children born are at or exceed the scores or measurements of those at the third percentile.

[43] Such an epicanthic fold is also typically seen in Down's syndrome or trisomy 21 (the presence of an extra, deleterious third twenty-first chromosome) babies, from which the previously common term of *Mongoloid idiot* derived—these children are also mentally retarded. It hardly needs to be said that the epicanthic folds of Orientals have an entirely different, genetic origin which has no reflection upon intelligence (if anything, Orientals, like Jews, tend to be rather smarter than other racial or ethnic groups). The epicanthic fold is thought to have developed in Asia in response to the extreme, bitter winter winds associated with the harsh conditions in Mongolia during the latter part of the Pleistocene glacial epoch.

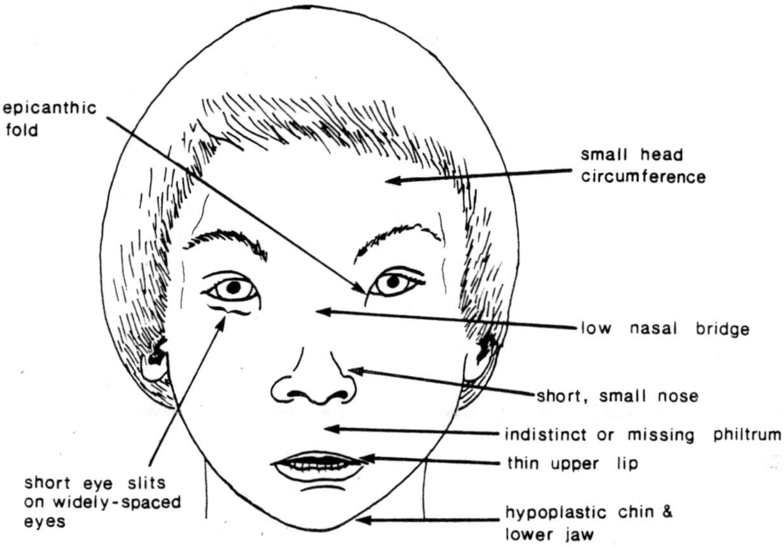

Figure 15. Facial Features of Fetal Alcohol Syndrome. After figures by Streissguth *et al.* 1980 and Sulik *et al.* 1981.

(b) a low nasal bridge and short nose and a long upper lip with an indistinct or entirely absent *philtrum*—the midmaxillary vertical groove running from beneath the nose to the upper border of the mouth. The red margin of the upper lip (*vermillion*) is characteristically extremely narrow. The forehead is typically narrow and the midface region flat and small; the lower jaw or *mandible* is often underdeveloped.

(4) Other associated features include (Streissguth *et al.* 1980):

(a) abnormal heart development, often with atrial or ventricular septal defects.

(b) abnormal development of the external genitalia.

(c) kidney abnormalities, including *hydronephrosis* or obstruction and distention of the kidneys with urine.

(d) restricted movement of the joints of the fingers and the elbows.

(e) abnormal palm crease patterns (this is also characteristic of Down's babies).

(f) weak sucking ability and other feeding problems, failure to thrive, delayed development, heightened sensitivity to sound, and diminished muscle tone.

A diagnosis of fetal alcohol syndrome generally requires the presence of the following minimal criteria (Chernoff 1980): (1) natal and postnatal growth retardation, (2) CNS functional abnormality, and (3) at least two of the major characteristic facial features of the syndrome discussed above. But even in the absence of the full syndrome a variety of adverse effects of alcohol upon intrauterine and postnatal growth and development have been demonstrated. The wide range of effects of alcohol upon fetal development are influenced by many factors: (1) the amount and duration of alcohol insult, (2) the specific stage(s) of fetal development in which the insult occurs, (3) the genetic and constitutional resistance of the fetus, and (4) in the case of animal models, the interspecific differences in vulnerability to FAS. Less than half of those alcoholic women who drink heavily throughout pregnancy bear FAS offspring, for example, and different strains of laboratory mice show different rates of malformation among their pups. Nevertheless, crude dose-response effects have been documented for FAS in both humans and animal models. The greater the intensity and duration of the onslaught, and the more vulnerable the stage of development at which the injury occurs, the greater, in general, will be the severity of FAS. Because one is dealing here with issues of degree and severity rather than of etiological difference, these lesser *teratogenic*[44] effects also represent manifestations of fetal alcohol syndrome.

Fetal alcohol effects can range from fullblown FAS in the offspring of chronic alcoholic women to a lower than average birth-weight in children born to women who drink an average of two to three drinks or more per day (Streissguth *et al.* 1980). Streissguth and her colleagues in a review of both the literature and their own data reported the following epidemiological statistics:

(1) a 32 percent prevalence of FAS babies among American chronic alcoholic mothers;

(2) a 33 percent prevalence for the full syndrome in the offspring of Swedish alcoholic mothers, and a 76 percent prevalence for partial fetal alcohol effects;

(3) a 26 percent frequency of FAS among the offspring of German alcoholic women—however, the rate was 43 percent among the severest alcoholic mothers and 20 percent for those with milder alcoholism.

(4) with regard to the prevalence of FAS in the general population, the following figures are reported: one severe case of FAS per 1000

[44] *Teratogenesis,* the development of gross structural fetal abnormalities, is multifactorial and is under both genetic and environmental influence. For example, the potent human teratogen thalidomide also produces severe malformations in several species of monkeys, but has no effect upon rats. Similarly, fetal alcohol abnormalities have been produced in fish, chickens, guinea pigs, and mice; dogs and rats do not appear to be as susceptible to fetal alcohol effects (Chernoff 1980).

births in northern France, but one in 400 when milder cases were also included; one in 600 births in Sweden and one in every 750 births in the United States show some characteristics of the fetal alcohol syndrome!

There appears to be a cross-cultural association between FAS and lower socioeconomic status, and recovered alcoholic American women of higher social and educational backgrounds show lower frequencies of FAS offspring resulting from pregnancies while they were still actively alcoholic (Streissguth *et al.* 1980). Smoking, poor nutrition, and other drug abuse may be contributing factors among lower socioeconomic FAS cases. It has been suggested (Streissguth *et al.* 1980; Mukherjee and Hodgen 1982) that an FAS prevalence of one out of every 750 births exists in the general population, which would make FAS one of the most common causes of mental retardation.

Several studies have shown that women who drink one to 1.6 ounces or more of alcohol per day during pregnancy have offspring weighing 59 to 169 grams less than do those who drink less (Streissguth *et al.* 1980). A French study (*loc. cit.*) revealed significantly different stillbirth rates of 9.9 per 1000 for light drinking mothers and 25.5 per 1000 for heavy drinkers. Heavy alcohol intake during pregnancy thus more than doubled the incidence of stillbirths; heavy drinking combined with smoking increased that rate more than five times (50.5 per 1000 births—Streissguth *et al.* 1980). Alcohol consumption during pregnancy is also associated with a *tenfold* increase in perinatal mortality (Sulik *et al.* 1981). Other studies (reported by Streissguth *et al.* 1980) revealed that the percentage of abnormal infants is directly related to the amount of maternal drinking: one study in Boston showed that 32 percent of the offspring of heavy drinking mothers had major or minor anomalies, as contrasted to 14 percent for moderate drinkers and nine percent for light drinking mothers. Early findings from an ongoing study (Dr. Paul M. Fernhof 1983, *in:* Family Practice News *13* (23): 1) show that of the offspring of moderate drinking mothers (60 ml or about 1.8 oz. of ethanol—two drinks—per day), 37 percent showed none, 47 percent had three or fewer, ten percent four to six, and seven percent exhibited more than seven of the features of FAS.

Other complicating factors such as smoking, greater age of the mother and higher number of previous viable offspring, lower socioeconomic class, and smoking were associated with even higher stillbirth rates. Genetic factors are also important and there are reports of dizygotic (fraternal) twins with differential expression of fetal alcohol effects from the same pregnancy (Streissguth *et al.* 1980). Because of differing individual susceptibilities to FAS *no safe maximal level of alcohol intake for all developing embryos can be proposed* (Chernoff 1980). Despite this, NIAAA[45] recommends a maximum of two drinks per day for pregnant women. As will become glaringly evident in the following paragraphs, the evidence strongly suggests that even one or two drinks *at any time* during pregnancy may have irreversible adverse effects on the developing fetus. The only possible conclusion is that pregnant women should refrain from *any* intake of alcohol or other drugs such as tobacco, caffeine, and even most over-the-counter or prescription drugs if at all possible.[46]

Variability in the expression of fetal alcohol effects also depends upon differences in the critial stages of embryogenesis at which alcohol insult occurs, the impacts of chronic versus binge drinking, and the maximum blood alcohol levels attained. Gross malformations are probably produced in the first trimester of pregnancy during development of the basic morphology of the central nervous system, whereas growth may be more vulnerable during the second and third trimesters (Figure 28). Behavior aberrations probably result from both early morphological anomalies in the CNS and the disruption of CNS functional organization during periods of rapid brain growth and differentiation (Rosett 1979). Such behavioral manifestations of fetal alcohol effects include decreased limb activity and increased amount of time spent with the eyes open and the head turned to the left than in control babies. Fundamental disturbances of basic regulatory devices are common in the offspring of alcoholic mothers—for example, sleep-wake cycles are typically disordered (*loc. cit.*).

In a recent study, Sulik and her colleagues (1981) demonstrated that even a brief exposure to alcohol on gestational day seven or eight in mice (corresponding to about the third week of human gestation) produces severe facial malformations very much like those seen in human FAS—including a narrow forehead, short palpebral fissures, small nose and midface region, and long upper lip with deficient or absent philtrum (see Figures 15 and 16). During this period of development, the *mesoderm* is

[45]National Institute on Alcohol Abuse and Alcoholism.

[46]Bendectin® (vitamin B_6 and antihistamine), despite the fact that it has been withdrawn from the market because of a landslide of unwarranted lawsuits, has been repeatedly documented as the only safe anti-nausea agent during pregnancy. Other over-the-counter drugs such as the aspirin substitute acetaminophen (Tylenol,® Datril,® Anacin-3®), most decongestants, and antacids (for pregnancy without renal dysfunction as a complicating factor) are also considered nonteratogenic and safe for the developing fetus.

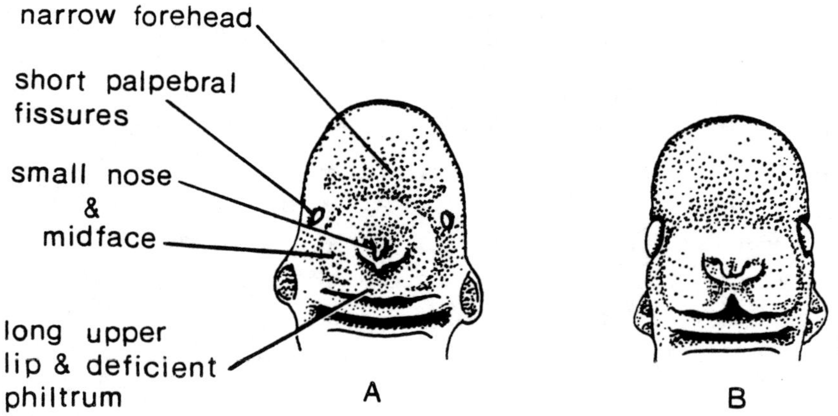

Figure 16. Effects of Ethanol on 14-Day-Old Mouse Fetuses. A. Alcohol-treated: two small doses administered to pregnant dam during the gastrulation stage of embryogenesis. **B.** Control. Gastrulation is the time of mesoderm formation, which is responsible for induction and maintenance of the neuroepithelium. These craniofacial malformations (A) are associated with gross histological abnormalities in the developing brain, including leptomeningeal neuroglial heterotopia (see also Figure 30). The disruption of mesoderm formation may underlie these changes. Drawn from figures by Sulik *et al.* 1981, Figure 1C-D. [See Figure 19.]

forming which induces the overlying *neuroectoderm* (see below) to differentiate first into a *neural plate* which then rolls up into an elongated *neural tube* (see Figure 20). The mesoderm is responsible for inducing and maintaining the formation of neural plate structures and their derivatives, particularly the evaginations of either side of the diencephalon (see Appendix 2) which form the retinal cup of the eye. The optic cup in turn induces the formation of the lens and other important structures of the eye which differentiate from the external *ectoderm* (see below). Teratogenic disruption of either the mesodermal structures or the neural plate can thus lead not only to gross CNS deformities but also to developmental anomalies of the eyes and associated organs.

Several studies have reported an abnormal migration of neural and glial cells[47] out onto the surface of the developing brain in human (Rosett 1979 and 1980; Streissguth *et al.* 1980) and mouse (Sulik *et al.* 1981) embryos exposed to alcohol (Figure 30). This condition, known as *leptomeningeal neuroglial heterotopia,* is associated with small brain size and other malformations (see also below). The doses of ethanol that produced the above facial changes and aberrant neural and glial sheets over the forebrain surface in mice were *two small doses administered four hours*

[47]Supportive, protective, and nutritive cells of the brain.

apart intraperitoneally on gestational day seven (Sulik *et al.* 1981)! Each pregnant female received 0.015 ml of ethanol per gram of body weight, and the blood alcohol concentration peaked at from 193 to 215 mg per ml (0.19 to 0.22%) some 20 to 25 minutes after administration; these blood alcohol levels fell to 30 mg per 100 ml within four hours.

These are very realistic blood alcohol levels for chronically alcoholic women. Furthermore, the very early period in embryogenesis at which these challenges were given correspond to about the third human gestational week, a point at which many women are not even yet aware that they are pregnant (Sulik *et al.* 1981). The incidence of fetal resorption in these ethanol treated mice was 18 percent relative to ten percent in controls and nearly 42 percent of the live fetuses had characteristic eye malformations. The clear implication is that even one or two episodes of heavy drinking early in the first trimester of pregnancy, a period when many women are unaware of being pregnant, may have disastrous effects upon the fetus.

Another study demonstrating the dramatic and potentially irreversible damage due to one or two single drinking episodes was recently carried out on monkeys (Mukherjee and Hodgen 1982). A single intravenous dose of ethanol given to pregnant rhesus monkeys caused a sudden and dramatic collapse of the entire umbilical vasculature within ten to 15 minutes after the challenge, with maximal effects at about 20 minutes. Gradual recovery from collapse began about 30 minutes after administration of the single dose and full recovery usually required about one hour. This collapse of the single umbilical vein[48] and the two umbilical arteries results in severe fetal hypoxia and acidosis, recovery coinciding with resumption of full fetal circulation in about one hour. Fetal blood *p*H values declined from 7.30 $\pm$ 0.08 at 15 minutes to 6.81 $\pm$ 0.05 at 30 minutes, and PO_2 values [49] from 38 $\pm$ 2 at time zero to 11 $\pm$ at 30 minutes. PCO_2 values varied from 40 $\pm$ 3 at time zero to 58 $\pm$ 5 at 30 minutes. Maternal blood alcohol concentrations peak at about

[48]See Figure 25 for a brief explanation of fetal circulation. The single large umbilical vein is a remnant of former paired umbilical veins. As the liver develops, the blood previously carried to the fetus by the right and proximal portion of the left umbilical veins is transported toward the heart via the liver sinuses, the hepatic vein and inferior vena cava, and these portions of the umbilical veins atrophy. The remaining distal portion of the left umbilical vein becomes very large and functions throughout fetal life to transport oxygenated blood from the placenta to the developing fetus.

[49]PO_2 and PCO_2 refer to the partial pressures of oxygen and carbon dioxide, respectively. The total pressure exerted by a mixture of gases under specified temperature and external pressure equals the sum of the partial pressures of the individual gases making up the mixture. The partial pressure of a gas is a direct measure of its relative concentration in the mixture.

250 ± 8.2 mg per 100 ml (0.25%) at 15 minutes and declined steadily afterwards; fetal blood alcohol levels peaked in about 30 minutes at only one-third that in the maternal circulation. An alcohol equilibrium between the fetal and maternal circulations was never achieved, and fetal blood alcohol clearance was a great deal slower than in the mothers. Acetaldehyde, on the other hand, reached peak and equilibrial values in both fetus and mother in 45 minutes and this equilibrium persisted after 75 minutes. Because of the low activity of fetal liver enzymes, the fetus may not be able to metabolize ethanol or acetaldehyde to any degree, and the clearance of both molecules from the fetal circulation may depend upon resumption of fetal circulation as the umbilical vasculature gradually recovers.[50]

The foregoing study by Mukherjee and Hodgen dramatically shows that a single strong challenge by ethanol to pregnant monkeys precipitates a sudden and complete, if temporary, loss of oxygenated blood to the fetus from the mother via the placenta. The resulting severe hypoxia to the fetal tissues is exacerbated by the fact that oxygen supply in the fetal circulation, and in particular to the developing CNS, is quite limited under the best of circumstances (see Figure 25). Such a temporary, though prolonged hypoxia may have severe consequences to the developing CNS during the first trimester of fetal growth. It would almost certainly have serious consequences later in pregnancy as the well-formed CNS undergoes rapid organization at increasingly complex levels. Oxygen starvation of as little as ten seconds in the adult human brain results in irreversible brain destruction. The evidence in animal models strongly suggests that acute, intermittent alcohol challenges to the developing fetus may be as deterimental as chronic ethanol insult throughout pregnancy. Although it remains unclear whether or not these observations can be extended to human beings, occasional or repeated binge drinking by pregnant alcoholic women in all likelihood produces severe hypoxia and acidosis in the developing fetus with potentially

[50]When the pregnant rats are given an ethanol challenge, only 25 percent of the acetaldehyde concentration in the peripheral maternal circulation is seen in the placenta and none appears in the fetal circulation (Rosett 1979; 1980). Because small molecules like ethanol and paraldehyde readily cross the placental barrier it is assumed that acetaldehyde is equally transportable into the fetal bloodstream, and it is likely that acetaldehyde is detoxified by the placental tissues. The situation with regard to human fetuses is unclear. Although most studies have assumed that acetaldehyde readily crosses the human placenta into the fetal circulation where it would cause even more damage than ethanol itself because of its higher toxicity (see for example, Pratt 1980; Lieber 1982), the case has not, in fact, been demonstrated. Human placental transfer and/or detoxification may or may not resemble the situation seen in monkeys reported above.

serious consequences for the CNS and neurological functioning (Rosett 1980).[51]

Acute hypoxia causes the breakdown of glucose into pyruvate and then into lactic acid in both the maternal and fetal circulations. The conversion of pyruvate into lactate is augmented by the elevated levels of reducing equivalents resulting from the oxidation of ethanol and acetaldehyde. [See Light 1985 for a discussion of alcohol-induced alterations of redox states.] With adequate glucose supplies, the lactic acid accumulation within the fetal brain cells may reach such levels that severe osmotic stress is placed upon the developing cerebral cells, and they may swell sufficiently to cause gross mechanical damage to the CNS (Pratt 1980). Lactic acid buildup in the fetus because of maternal alcohol intake has been documented in both human beings (Pratt 1980) and animal models (Rosett 1980).

The fetal liver lacks *phosphoenolpyruvate carboxykinase,*[52] the enzyme which converts oxaloacetate into phosphoenolpyruvate (PEP), the first step in gluconeogenesis. The fetus is thus unable to synthesize glucose, and any episode of ethanol-induced hypoglycemia in the maternal circulation (see Light 1985) can result in a profound fall of fetal blood glucose levels (Pratt 1980). Since fetal blood glucose levels are normally less than in the maternal circulation, the hypoglycemia induced in the fetus can be severe. The fetal brain is almost totally dependent upon glucose for normal functioning. Any drop in fetal blood glucose concentrations results in a corresponding decrease in the transfer of glucose across the fetal blood-brain barrier. A glucose insufficiency may adversely affect dividing and migrating brain cells in the developing fetus, and may underlie many of the malformations and functional impairment of the CNS seen in FAS (Pratt 1980). The threat of a severe hypoglycemic episode in a pregnant, binge-drinking, alcoholic woman is a very real one (see Light 1985).

Advanced liver cirrhosis in alcoholic women generally results in such massive endocrine dysfunction, including *amenorrhea* (complete cessation of the menstrual cycle), that pregnancy rarely occurs. Nevertheless,

[51]Hypoxia can result in the breakdown of glucose to pyruvate and lactate in the advanced fetal brain (Pratt 1980). Even in the absence of hypoxia, alcohol intoxication generates excessive blood concentrations of lactate because of the drastically altered redox balance (see Light 1985). Such lactic acidosis in a pregnant woman would inevitably cause a similar acidosis within the fetus, and CNS damage would be a very likely consequence.

[52]Also termed *phosphoenolpyruvate carboxylase.* This enzyme is necessary to sidestep the energetic barrier between pyruvate and phosphoenolpyruvate to initiate gluconeogenesis. (See Light 1985 for a detailed discussion of carbohydrate metabolism.)

liver damage in pregnant women represents a very real threat to the survival and well-being of the fetus. Alcohol insult during pregnancy contributes to fetal as well as maternal hepatic dysfunction (Rosett 1980; Pratt 1980), and the hepatic cells of rat pups born to dams which had been fed ethanol during pregnancy showed gross enlargement and disruption of the mitochondria (Beskid *et al.* 1975 *in* Rosett 1980). Hepatic microsomal enzymes (cytochrome P-450, see Light 1985), appear to be induced in both the fetus and the mother by ethanol challenges, and a buildup of reducing equivalents consequent to alcohol metabolism is seen in both the pregnant dam and fetus. Several studies have shown that protein synthesis is significantly depressed in both maternal and fetal livers in response to maternal alcohol consumption. High doses of ethanol also reduce protein synthesis in maternal kidney and placental as well as fetal heart and kidney tissues (Henderson *et al.* 1980 *in* Rosett 1980).

Maternal and fetal liver injury is associated with enhanced plasma levels of aromatic amino acids, whereas the branched-chain amino acids (leucine, isoleucine and valine) are significantly depressed. This increased ratio of aromatic to branched-chain amino acids results in enhanced transport of the former across the blood-brain barrier into the CNS.[53] Several authors have proposed that this enhanced ratio of aromatic amino acids is at least partially responsible for hepatic encephalopathy (see Light 1985). The increased concentration of aromatic amino acids could lead to the production of a variety of false transmitters in the brain, thus contributing to CNS dysfunction (Lieber 1982; however, this author notes several recent reports that challenge this hypothesis). The deficit of branched-chain amino acids may directly result in brain damage since they are essential to the metabolism of protein within the brain (Pratt 1980). Cerebral protein is constantly being synthesized and degraded and the branched-chain amino acids play a vital role in this process. The normal metabolic pathways of central neurotransmitters are also very likely to be disrupted by such abnormal amino acid balances. The same displacement of amino acids on common carrier proteins described for the blood-brain barrier also applies to the placental barrier, and altered concentrations of amino acids in the maternal circulation would very likely be reflected in the fetal circulation.[54]

[53]The greater concentration of aromatic amino acids results in a competitive advantage for binding sites on the common carrier proteins relative to the branched-chain fraction.

[54]Heavy-drinking pregnant women have placentas weighing on the average 22 grams less than those of lighter drinkers (Rosett 1980).

Protein synthesis in the livers of fetal and neonatal rats of dams challenged by ethanol during pregnancy is significantly reduced relative to controls. In particular, leucine, one of the branched-chain amino acids, was incorporated into protein to a significantly smaller extent, perhaps reflecting the general depression in the levels of such amino acids in response to maternal alcohol intake (Rosett 1980). This inhibition of protein synthesis appears to be directly related to retarded fetal growth in the offspring of alcoholic dams. Even *hypothermia* (lowered body temperature) produced in the mother because of ethanol-induced peripheral vasodilation and depression of the hypothalmic temperature-regulating centers contributes to reduced rates of protein synthesis.

A variety of vitamin and mineral deficiencies are associated with chronic alcoholism because of inadequate diet, impaired intestinal uptake and increased *diuresis* (urinary output),[55] diarrhea and vomiting. The consumption of 30 ml of ethanol by normal volunteers results in a 100 percent increase in urinary excretion of calcium and a 167 percent increase in the excretion of magnesium (Rosett 1980). Lowered serum levels and increased urinary excretion of magnesium and zinc are commonly seen among alcoholic humans, whereas serum copper concentrations and liver iron stores appear to be increased (Mendelson and Huber 1980). It has been suggested that some of the abnormalities associated with fetal alcohol syndrome may be related to altered mineral and trace element metabolism in the mother and developing fetus. Both magnesium and zinc deficiencies alone produce a variety of congenital malformations in rats. A recent study by Mendelson and Huber (1980) showed that alcohol challenges to pregnant rats without mineral supplements results in significant reduction of magnesium and zinc deposition in maternal femurs[56]; this effect was overcome by the addition of these minerals to the diet. The fetuses in the alcohol-treated groups showed no reduction in magnesium deposition, but exhibited a moderate decrease in zinc deposition which was eliminated by the addition of zinc to the diet. However, the degree of reduced deposition of these minerals was not sufficient to account for the birth defects associated with such deficiences.

The following description of human development is largely distilled from Arey 1965 and Moore 1977. Development or embryogenesis begins

[55] See Light 1986a. Alcohol inhibits the production of vasopressin (antidiuretic hormone) in the posterior pituitary, thus increasing urinary output.

[56] The femur conserves trace elements and does not respond to transient fluctuations of these substances.

when the ovum is fertilized by a spermatozoan. Once the mature ovum is released from the ovary, it is capable of fertilization for 12 to 24 hours. The spermatozoa can remain viable for about 24 to 72 hours following ejaculation into the female reproductive tract. All sorts of obstacles impede their survival, including acidic fluids in the vagina and exhaustion from the long, vigorous trip up into the fallopian tubules, and the mortality is very high. Of the half billion or so spermatozoa contained in a single ejaculate, perhaps but a few hundred thousand actually survive to enter the fallopian tubules. When the sperm encounter the ovum, they release certain enzymes, in particular *hyaluronidase,* which dissolve the follicle cells surrounding the ovum, allowing the spermatozoa to penetrate to the surface of the egg. When a single spermatozoan encounters the egg itself, it fuses with the outer membrane of the egg, and in a complex process is drawn inside the cytoplasm of the ovum. At the instant of fertilization, the spermatozoan sheds its motile "tail," and the cell membrane of the ovum and an outer, noncellular layer membrane called the *zona pellucida* undergo expansion and transformation such that all other spermatozoa are excluded. This ensures that only one spermatozoan will fertilize the egg, so that the normal human chromosome complement of 46 chromosomes will result. The fertilized egg undergoes its final reduction (meiotic) divisions and is now known as a *zygote.* Figure 17 illustrates these events and briefly describes the ensuing processes of early *cleavage* and *implantation.*

Cleavage proceeds until a hollow sphere of cells known as the *blastocyst* is formed (Figures 17D and 18A). Attached to one side of the inner surface of this hollow ball is a small group of cells called the *inner cell mass* (Figures 17D and 18A), from which the embryo itself will develop. The layer of cells forming the hollow ball is called the *trophoblast* and the cavity it contains is known as the *blastocoel* (Figure 18A). Implantation within the uterine wall occurs between days six and nine following fertilization; blastocysts which do not become implanted undergo spontaneous abortion or miscarriage and are expelled out the vagina.

Shortly after implantation, a cavity forms within the proliferating inner cell mass (Figure 18B). This *amniotic cavity* separates that portion of the inner cell mass destined to become the future embryo from the trophoblast. The membrane surrounding the amniotic cavity is called the *amnion*; the amnion will eventually expand enormously to surround the entire fetus in a protective, fluid-filled sac (see Figures 20, 22 and 23). Those cells of the former inner cell mass that lie on the floor of the amniotic cavity and which project farthest into the blastocoel comprise

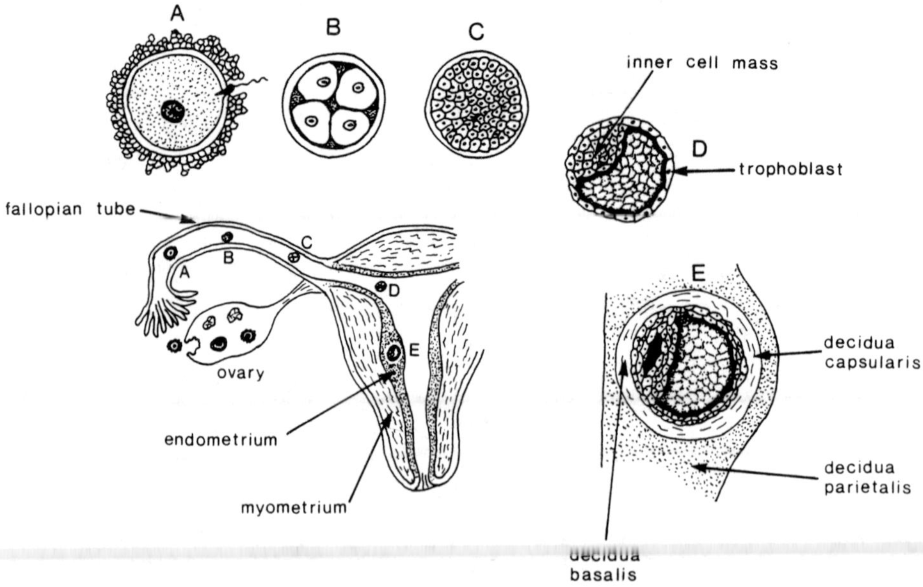

Figure 17. Fertilization, Cleavage, and Implantation. Ovulation involves the rupturing of the Graafian follicle and release of the egg or ovum from the ovary. The egg then enters the fallopian tube where fertilization with a spermatozoan (A) occurs within one to two days of ovulation while the ovum is still fairly high in the fallopian tube. The fertilized egg or zygote immediately begins to divide (B) into two cells or blastomeres, which in turn cleave into four cells, then eight, and so on until a hollow ball made up of many cells, the blastocyst (D), is formed. The blastocyst then becomes implanted (E) in the uterine mucosa or endometrium, where subsequent development occurs. That portion of the endometrium lying between the implanted blastocyst and the outer muscular wall of the uterus or myometrium is called the decidua basalis. Together with tissues from the developing embryo, it will form the placenta. That part of the endometrium between the embryo and the uterine cavity is the decidua capsularis, and the remainder of the endometrium is known as the decidua parietalis.

the *embryonic disc.* These are the cells from which the embryo itself will develop. The layer of cells immediately adjacent to the amniotic cavity is known as the *epiblast*; it will give rise to the *ectoderm*—the germ layer from which the skin, nervous system, bones of the skull and face, and other specialized tissues are derived. The layer of cells adjacent to the blastocoel will give rise to the *endoderm*—that germ layer giving rise to the viscera and their derivatives. The middle germ layer or *mesoderm* in humans is derived both extraembryonically from the trophoblast and intraembryonically from ingressing ectodermal cells during the process of *gastrulation* (see below, and Figures 18 and 19).

At the time of implantation (gestational day six to seven) the trophoblast differentiates into an outer *syncytial trophoblast* and an inner

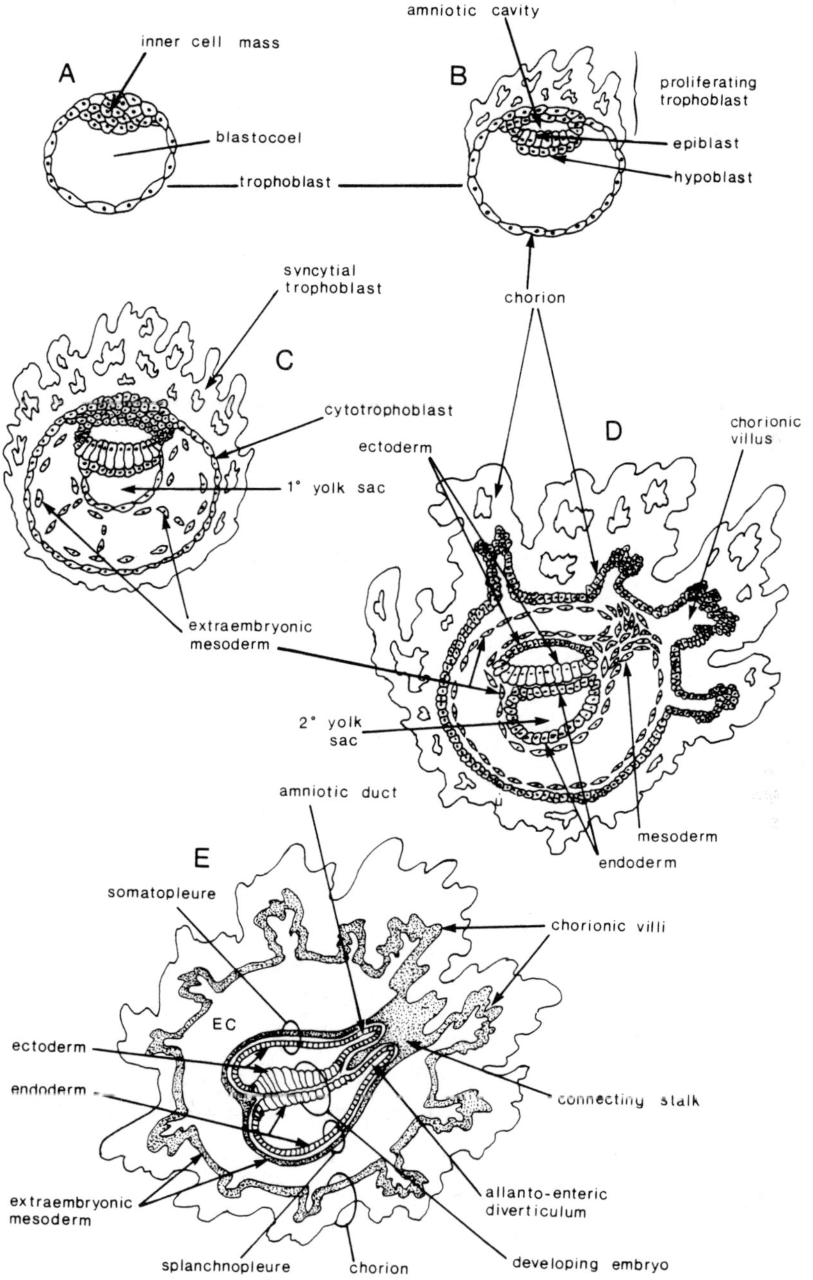

Figure 18. Early Formation of the Embryo and Extraembryonic Membranes. A. Human blastocyst at six days. **B.** Partially implanted blastocyst, about eight days. [The endometrium is not shown in this figure.] **C.** Fully implanted blastocyst of about nine days. **D.** Implanted human embryo at about 14 days. **E.** Human embryo at a slightly later stage. The transient amniotic duct has formed as has the allantoenteric diverticulum, but the embryo is still at the bilaminar (two-layered) stage, and the primitive streak and primitive knot have not yet formed. See text for details. EC = extraembryonic coelom.

layer known as the *cytotrophoblast* (Figure 18C). The syncytial trophoblast (syncytiotrophoblast) is an erosive, non-cellular, multinucleated tissue[57] which aggressively invades the *decidua basalis* of the uterine wall (Figures 17E and 18C-E). As the trophoblast invades the uterine wall, nutrients are derived from the digested tissues and the blastocyst becomes more and more deeply implanted within the endometrium. The cytotrophoblast undergoes rapid cell division which supply the proliferating syncytiotrophoblast. Other cells delaminate from the cytotrophoblast into the blastocoel to form a thin layer of *extraembryonic* (derived from outside the embryo itself) *mesoderm,* also known as *Heuser's membrane* (Figure 18C-D).

The bilaminar trophoblast (cytotrophoblast and syncytiotrophoblast together) forms the *chorion.* In the region of the decidua basalis the chorion produces a number of complex fingerlike processes which penetrate still deeper into the uterine wall. These processes are the *chorionic villi* (Figure 18D-E). Branches of the developing umbilical arteries and vein[58] invade the chorionic villi and form complex capillary networks. Isolated spaces or *lacunae* appear in the syncytiotrophoblast (see Figure 18D) at about day nine which become filled with maternal blood from the eroded endometrium (decidua basalis). Uterine vessels then join with these lacunae to initiate uteroplacental circulation. The *placenta* is thus formed of both fetal (chorionic villi) and maternal (decidua basalis) tissues (see Figures 17, 18 and 24). The maternal and fetal circulations are separated by the fetal chorion and capillary *endothelium* (cells lining the capillary walls) and there is usually no intermingling of the two blood supplies.[59] However, small molecules such as gases (oxygen, carbon dioxide), glucose, amino acids, fats and other nutrients readily move across this *placental barrier* and provide for nutrition and removal of metabolic wastes from the fetus.

The chorionic villi first appear during gestational days 13 to 14 and the essential structure and function of the primitive uteroplacental circulation, that is, the physiological exchanges between the embryo and the mother, are operational by the beginning of the fourth week of development. Chorionic villi develop over the entire surface of the chorion until

[57] A *syncytium* is a tissue containing many nuclei in which no cell boundaries are discernible; normally there is but one nucleus per cell.

[58] The single umbilical vein represents a fusion of two precursor umbilical veins.

[59] A very small amount of mixing does occur because of small ruptures that appear in both the fetal and maternal capillaries. This can cause serious problems in subsequent pregnancies when Rh factors are incompatible between the mother and the fetus.

about week eight. Thereafter the villi associated with the decidua capsularis (see Figure 22) atrophy and disappear and the entire growth of the chorion becomes focused in the region of the decidua basalis. This region of the chorion is then known as the *villous chorion* or the *chorion frondosum.* The maternal component of the placenta arises from the decidua basalis. As the chorionic villi invade the decidua basalis, a number of wall-like septa remain in the spaces between the advancing villi (Figures 22 and 24). The lacunae which appeared earlier in the syncytiotrophoblast become enlarged into interconnecting *intervillous spaces.* These, in turn, are penetrated by a complex network of maternal (uterine) arteries and veins which transport essential substances to the fetus via the placenta and fetal waste products from the placenta. The mature placenta is illustrated in Figure 24.

The delaminating cells of the extraembryonic mesoderm come to surround the developing embryo as well as line the entire inner surface of the chorion, thus forming a completely mesoderm-lined *extraembryonic coelom* (Figures 18E and 22). The layer of extraembryonic mesoderm that overlies the hypoblast of the embryonic disc lift off to form a hollow *primary yolk sac* (Figure 18C). Soon afterward, the hypoblastic (endodermal) cells migrate downward to cover the inner surface of the extraembryonic mesodermal cells forming the primary yolk sac. The extraembryonically derived primary yolk sac then atrophies and disappears in a as yet poorly understood process, leaving behind a *secondary yolk sac* formed of embryonic endodermal cells and covered on the outside by extraembryonic mesoderm (Figure 18D). This secondary yolk sac will persist for a while and give rise to the primitive precursors of the circulatory system.

As mentioned in the foregoing paragraph, the extraembryonic coelom[60] is completely lined with extraembryonically derived mesoderm. Ectodermal cells from the epiblastic layer grow upward to cover the inner surface of the amnion (Figures 18D-E, 19 and 22). This double membrane is referred to as the *somatopleure* and the mesoderm associated with it is the *somatic mesoderm.* The somatopleure will form the outer wall of the true coelom or body cavity of the fetus. A transient structure, the *amniotic duct,* briefly penetrates into the *connecting stalk* or future *umbilicus* which connects the embryo to the chorion. The amniotic duct soon disappears and its function is not known.

The secondary yolk sac is also contained within a bilayer called the *splanchnopleure.* The splanchnopleure consists of endoderm which grows

[60]The coelom is defined as a body cavity which is completely lined with mesoderm.

downward from the hypoblast and an outer layer of *splanchnic mesoderm* (Figures 18D-E and 19). The viscera, including the lungs, stomach, gut, pancreas, liver and other organs will develop from the endoderm. The splanchnic mesoderm will line the inner surface of the true coelom and will form the *mesenteries,* the sheets of connective tissue which enclose the visera and which suspend them in the coelom from the outer body wall. An outpocketing of the posterior yolk sac known as the *allantoenteric diverticulum* (Figures 18E and 19) extends into the connecting stalk. This structure does not disappear but develops into the *allantois* which is destined to participate in the formation of the bladder and associated structures. The yolk sac and allantois, together with the chorion will initiate the development of the circulatory system.

The chorion, amnion, yolk sac and the allantois are known as the *extraembryonic membranes.* They develop from, but do not form parts of the embryo itself, except that portions of the yolk sac are incorporated into the gut lining and part of the allantois remains as a ligament extending from the urinary bladder to the umbilicus. These membranes along with the placenta (also partially an extraembryonic structure) provide for protection and support, nutrition, respiration and excretion for the fetus. They are expelled from the uterus as the *afterbirth* when the baby is born.

By gestational day 15, a thickened, longitudinal band known as the *primitive streak* appears in the posterior midline of the epiblast (Figure 19). The primitive streak grows longer by adding cells at its posterior end. As it grows forward along the embryonic disc, a *primitive groove* forms in the primitive streak, and a thickened mass of cells, the *primitive knot,* appears at the anterior end. The primitive groove is confluent with a depression in the primitive knot called the *primitive pit.* These cells invaginate over the lip of the primitive groove and pit and penetrate between the overlying epiblast, now called the ectoderm, and the hypoblast, now called the endoderm (Figures 18, 19A, and 20A-B). These cells migrate laterally and anteriorly to form an intermediate layer, the *intraembryonic mesoderm* (Figures 19A and 20C).

At about day 16 a group of cells migrates forward from the primitive knot to form a median rodlike structure known as the *head process* or *notochordal process* (Figure 20A-D). This rodlike structure will form the *notochord,* the primitive precursor of the spinal column seen in all vertebrates. The head process grows anteriorly only as far as a point of fusion between the anterior ectoderm and endoderm (see Figure 20A, not labelled). This point of fusion between the ectoderm and endoderm will eventually give

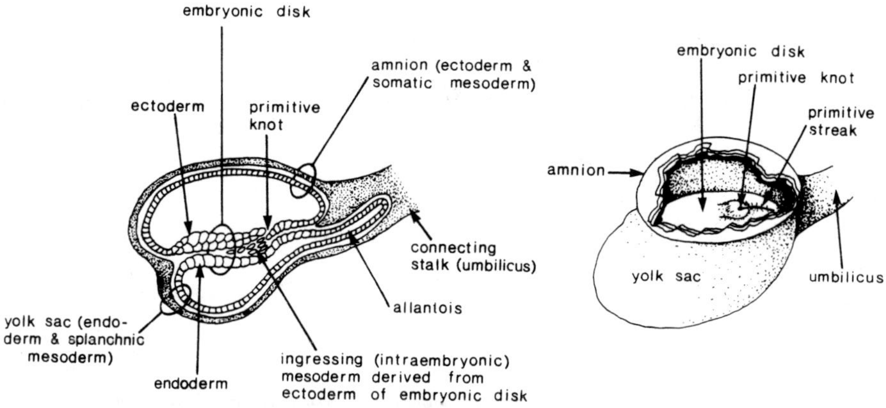

Figure 19. Gastrulating Human Embryo. A. Section through a 16-day-old gastrulating human embryo showing the relationships between the embryonic disc, the three germ layers—ectoderm, mesoderm, and endoderm, and the fetal membranes. **B.** Three-dimensional view of the same stage through a cut-away portion of the amnion, showing the embryonic disc, the primitive streak and the primitive knot from which the ingressing intraembryonic mesoderm derives. Redrawn from a figure by Arey 1965.

rise to the *oropharyngeal membrane* (Figure 22), which will eventually rupture to form the *stomodaeum* where the ectoderm of the mouth joins the endoderm of the foregut.

The notochord is often referred to as the *primary inducer.* The very presence of this rodlike structure *induces* the immediately overlying ectoderm to differentiate into a *neural plate* (Figure 20B-C). The ectoderm of the neural plate, the *neuroectoderm,* will give rise to the brain, spinal cord and derived structures. At about day 18 the neural plate gives rise to two longitudinal *neural folds* (Figure 20D). These folds converge and fuse medially to form a closed *neural tube* (Figure 20E-F), which will differentiate into the various regions of the brain and spinal cord (see Appendix 2 and Light 1986a for subsequent development of the CNS). When the neural tube closes sequentially along its length (see Figure 20F), certain neuroectodermal cells on either side of the neural plate are pinched off. These cells, the *neural crest cells* (Figure 20D), will migrate to all parts of the developing body to form the entire peripheral nervous system and a variety of other structures, including the *melanocytes* or pigment cells of the skin, the *chromaffin cells* of the adrenal medulla, and even cartilage.

The ingressing extraembryonic mesoderm on either side of the notochord forms a flat, sheetlike mass which becomes differentiated into longitudinal columns of *paraxial mesoderm* lying immediately adjacent to the notochord on each side. The paraxial mesoderm will give rise to

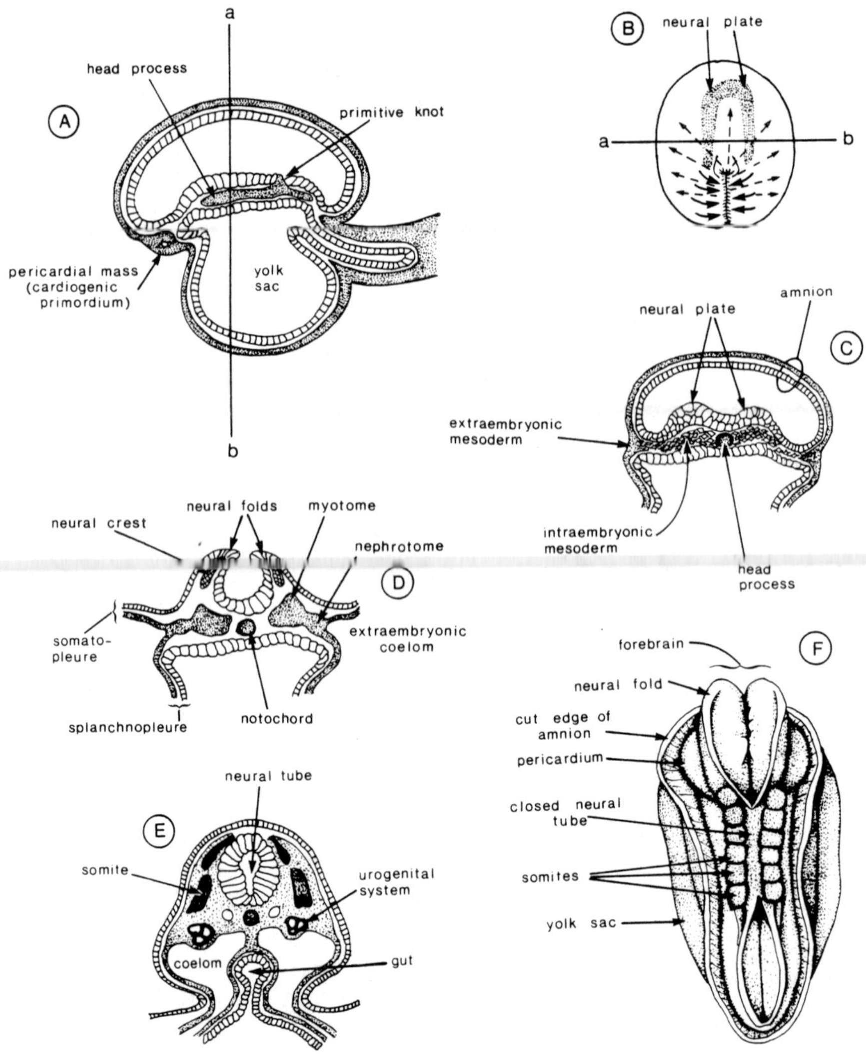

Figure 20. Six-Somite Stage (About Three Weeks). A. Longitudinal section through embryonic disc and extraembryonic membranes (amnion and yolk sac). Embryonically derived mesoderm from the primitive streak area has invaded between the overlying ectoderm and underlying endoderm. This forward projecting mesoderm is known as the head process; it gives rise to and is indistinguishable from the notochord—the primary organizer for all subsequent development and which gives rise to the future spinal column. Line a to b in both A and B show the plane of sections C to E. **B.** View of 16-day-old embryonic disc from above showing the primitive streak and knot and the developing neural plate which gives rise to the neural folds (see C to E), and ultimately, to the neural tube. Solid arrows show epiboly and the movement of cells toward the primitive streak for invagination into the interior; hatched-line arrows show the direction of movement of invaginated mesoderm lying between the ectoderm and endoderm. **C.** Cross-section through A, showing neural plate induced by the notochord. The intraembryonic mesoderm has fused laterally with the extraembryonic mesoderm. **D.** A somewhat later stage (about 21 days). →

some 38 pairs or so of serial, cuboidal *somites* (Figure 20D-F) which give rise to specific muscles, skeletal vertebrae and other structures. As can be seen from Figure 20F, the serially arranged somites represent a sequence of repetitive segments, that is, the vertebrate embryo exhibits segmentation or *metamerism.* Immediately lateral to the paraxial mesoderm is the *intermediate mesoderm.* The intermediate mesoderm gives rise to the serial *nephrotomes* associated with each somite (Figure 20D). The nephrotome eventually will give rise to the urogenital system in a series of stages too complex to describe here. The intermediate mesoderm merges with the *lateral plate mesoderm* which, in turn, fuses with the extraembryonic mesoderm (Figure 20C-D).

Blood vessels begin to form during days 13 to 15. They first appear in the splanchnic mesoderm of the yolk sac, connecting stalk and chorion as isolated *blood islands* or masses of cells in which spaces appear. These blood islands become differentiated into elongated cords, and as the spaces within these masses become more extensive, primitive blood vessels appear. Some of the cells lining the spaces give rise to the first blood cells floating in a primitive blood plasma secreted by these same cells. These isolated vessels coalesce into a capillary network which progressively invade the embryo. At the same time, intraembryonic vessels begin to appear throughout the embryonic mesoderm as they are needed, and as these vessels merge with the extraembryonic ones the primitive circulatory system is established. Blood cells are successively formed from: the yolk sac (week four), embryonic mesenchyme and blood vessels (week five), the liver (week six), spleen, thymus and lymphatic system (second to fourth months) and thereafter in the bone marrow (Arey 1965).

In a similar way, the paired primitive *heart tubes* differentiate out of the *cardiogenic primordium* (Figure 20A) during the third week of development. These two vessels will soon differentiate into the paired *aortic*

The neural folds are well developed and are beginning to roll overhead to form the neural tube. Neural crest cells are now well differentiated; these will eventually split off to form a variety of cells and tissue types in the adult (peripheral ganglia, portions of the endocrine system, etc.). The lateral plate mesoderm has differentiated into the serial somites on either side of the notochord; the nephrotome, which will give rise to the urogenital system, has already begun to differentiate. The extraembryonic coelom is lined with mesoderm derived from three sources: somatic mesoderm associated with the amniotic ectoderm, splanchnic mesoderm associated with the endoderm of the yolk sac, and extraembryonic mesoderm derived from the syncytiotrophoblast (see also Figure 18). **E.** Cross-section of later stage (26 days) with completely formed neural tube; the gut is beginning to form from the endoderm. **F.** Overhead view of a six-somite state.

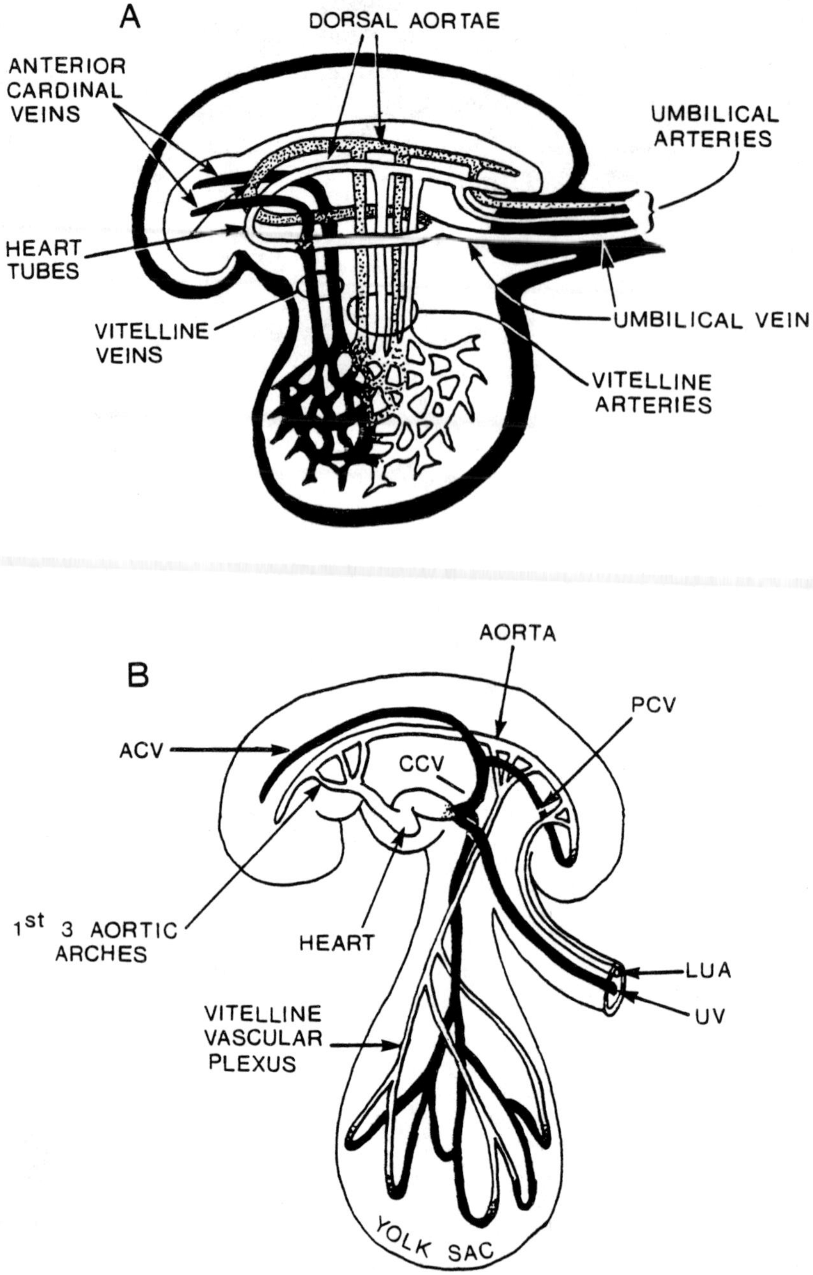

Figure 21. The Early Cardiovascular System. A. 21-day-old human embryo. Blood vessel formation begins in the extraembryonic mesoderm of the yolk sac, connecting stalk and chorion during the third week. *Blood islands* first form around lacunae peripheral to the embryonic disc; these then invade the embryo itself. Paired *heart tubes* develop from the *cardiogenic primordium* (Figure 20A) and merge with the paired *dorsal aortae* which carry blood posteriorly from the heart. The paired umbilical arteries and the single *umbilical vein* →

arches and the paired *dorsal aortae* (Figure 21); ventromedially the two heart tubes fuse into the single primitive heart. The aortic arches are the evolutionary homologues[61] of the gill arches of fishes. They will differentiate into the major arteries of the head and thorax (see Figure 25) and some will atrophy and disappear altogether. The transient *vitelline arteries* and the *umbilical arteries* arise from the paired dorsal aortae. By the fourth week the dorsal aortae will have fused into the single *descending aorta* over much of their lengths (Figure 25). By this time also the paired *precardinal, postcardinal* and *common cardinal veins,* and the paired *vitelline umbilical veins* have appeared (Figure 21). The vitelline circulation bringing blood to and from the yolk sac lasts for only a very short time and these vessels soon disappear. The paired umbilical veins will fuse into a single vessel which will persist throughout development to bring oxygen and nutrients from the placenta to the fetus.[62] Portions of the cardinal and umbilical veins are destined to give rise to the *superior* (anterior) and *inferior* (posterior) *venae cavae,* the *hepatic portal vein,* and the transient embryonic umbilical vein and the *ductus venosus* (Figure 25). The paired posterior cardinal veins will form the vasculature of the urogenital system. The circulatory system is the first fully functional one to develop in the fetus.

The fourth to eighth weeks of embryogenesis are very critical ones. The development of all major organ systems is initiated during this

[61]Structures in different organisms having the same evolutionary derivatives.

[62]Spent, deoxygenated blood is carried from the fetus to the placenta by the paired umbilical arteries.

(originally formed from paired vessels) carry blood to and from the placenta, respectively. The *vitelline arteries* lead from the dorsal aortae to a vascular plexus in the yolk sac, and the *vitelline veins* return it to the heart tubes. The *anterior cardinal veins* (ACV) return spent blood from the head. Both sides of these paired systems are shown. **B.** 26-day-old embryo, vessels of left side only. The two heart tubes have fused into the primitive heart, which receives spent blood from the paired ACV and *posterior cardinal veins* (PCV) via the *common cardinal veins* (CCV), which in turn empty into the posterior part of the heart via the *sinus venosus* (Figure 25). Portions of the PCV will form the *hepatic portal vein* and part of the *inferior vena cava.* As development proceeds, the sinus venosus shifts to the right and eventually drains into what will become the right auricle. The left ACV becomes the left *brachiocephalic vein* and the right ACV and right CCV become the *superior vena cava.* During the fourth week *aortic arches* form from the anterior heart region (truncus arteriosus); six arches will eventually develop, but they are not all present at the same time. They are homologous with the gill arches of lower vertebrates (see footnotes 66 and 77). Some of these arches become several important anterior arteries of the adult circulation, and some merely atrophy and disappear. LUA = left umbilical artery; UV = umbilical vein. Cf. Figure 25.

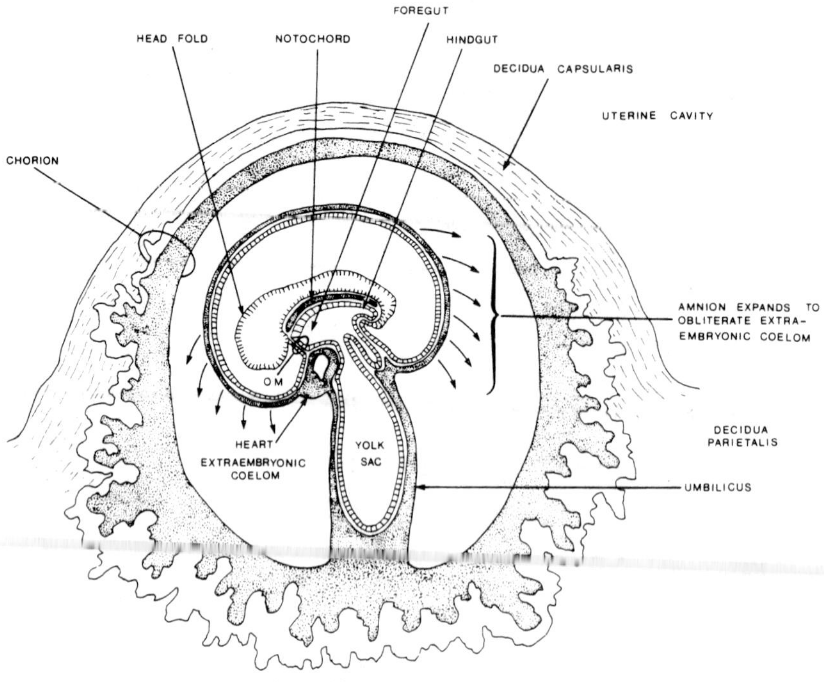

Figure 22. Human Embryo at 26 Days. The pericardial region is well developed from the area below the head where the somatic and splanchnic mesoderm fused earlier (see Figure 18). The oropharyngeal membrane (OM) has formed from the fusion of the embryonic ectoderm and endoderm just anterior to the forward extension of the notochord (head process) [see also Figure 20]. As the embryo folds inward still further to incorporate the developing heart inside the body (note the expanding amnion), the oropharyngeal membrane will rupture to form the mouth and pharynx. The foregut and hindgut are well advanced; the yolk sac will ultimately degenerate, but remnants will form the single umbilical vein and the paired umbilical arteries which connect the fetus with the placenta (see also Figure 23). The amnion is rapidly expanding in all directions. It will eventually completely obliterate the extraembryonic coelom, except for that portion which becomes pinched off by the amniotic folds (Figure 20E) and incorporated inside the fetus to form the true body cavity or coelom. The inner surface of this coelom is lined by splanchnopleure and the outer surface by somatopleure. Within this cavity the body organs are suspended by mesodermally derived sheets of tissue—the mesenteries. In this figure, the chorionic villi have already disappeared from most of the chorion except for that portion attached to the decidua basalis. In that region the villi become even more extensive and together with the maternal decidua, form the placenta (see Figure 24).

period. It is during this time, also, that exposure of the embryo to *teratogens,*[63] such as alcohol and other drugs, can result in major congenital deformities (Figure 28). The three-layered embryo has become an elongated, cylindrical one. The rapidly growing forebrain region projects

---

[63]Any agent or substance capable of causing congenital malformations.

anteriorly beyond the area of the oropharyngeal membrane (Figure 22) as an overhanging *head fold.* A similar overgrowth of the posterior neural tube results in an overhanging *tail fold* (shown, but not labelled in Figure 22). This differential anterior and posterior growth causes the developing heart region and the forward and rear portions of the yolk sac to fold inward and upward onto the ventral part of the embryo. These folded portions of the yolk sac thus become incorporated into the embryo as the fore- and hindgut regions. The foregut comes to lie between the forebrain and the heart region and it terminates at the oropharyngeal membrane which will ultimately rupture to form the mouth.

In addition to this *longitudinal folding, transverse folding* also occurs at this time. The outer body wall region (somatopleure) folds inward towards the midline of the embryo (Figure 20E; shown but not labelled) to form lateral and ventral walls enclosing what has now become the *intraembryonic coelom.*[64] The embryo is now attached to the extraembryonic yolk sac by a narrow passage in the midbody region. At the same time the amnion expands completely away from the embryo (Figure 22) and eventually obliterates the remaining extraembryonic coelom completely. In so doing it fuses with the chorion and envelops and fuses with the former connecting stalk (Figure 23), forming what is now called the *umbilical cord.* The remaining part of the yolk sac lying outside the embryo will atrophy and disappear.

The primitive axial support in all vertebrates is the notochord. In very primitive chordates like *Amphioxus,* the larvae of tunicates,[65] and in primitive jawless vertebrates like the lampreys and hagfishes, the notochord provides the entire skeletal support. In all higher vertebrates (from the fishes on up), however, the notochord is replaced during embryonic development by a cartilaginous or bony axial skeleton. Most of the spinal column in mammals is derived from portions of the serial somites which differentiate into the various parts of the vertebrae. This region of the somites, known as the *sclerotome* (not figured here), migrates dorso- and ventromedially to enclose the developing neural tube

[64]Actually cavities begin to open up within the embryo proper by a splitting of the lateral plate mesoderm (not figured here). These intraembryonic spaces also separate an outer somatopleure from an inner splanchnopleure, and much of the intraembryonic coelom is derived from these spaces. In the midbody region the intraembryonic cavities communicate freely with the extraembryonic coelom. As the lateral folds enclose the embryo ventrally, portions of the former extraembryonic coelom become incorporated inside the embryo and together with the intraembryonically derived body cavity form the coelom of the fetus.

[65]Members of the phylum Chordata, to which we belong, are characterized by having, among other things, a notochord at least sometime during their life cycle. Tunicates or "sea squirts" belong to the subphylum Urochordata. They possess a notochord during their free-swimming, tadpolelike larval stage. The sessile adults are colonial and resemble encrusting sponges.

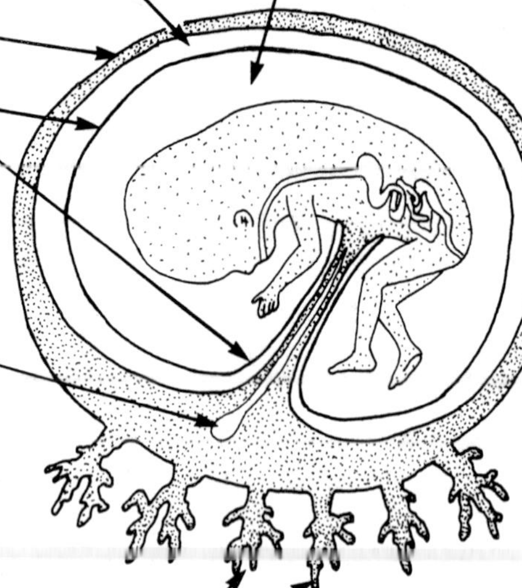

Figure 23. Human Fetus at About 11 Weeks. The extraembryonic coelom is all but obliterated, the visera are completely contained within the body cavity formed by extraembryonic remnants enveloped by the folds of the aminon as they enclose the embryo ventrally and laterally (see Figure 20). The umbilicus is now contained within the following membranes from the inside out: yolk sac endoderm and its associated extraembryonic splanchnic mesoderm, both forming the splanchnopleure, and extraembryonic somatic mesoderm and its associated extraembryonic (amniotic) ectoderm, both forming the somatopleure.

within a bony, protective arch so that the spinal cord is contained within the bony elements of the spinal column. Only remnants of the notochord persist as part of the *intervertebral discs* which separate and cushion the vertebrae. Other regions of the somites, the *myotome,* develop into the heavy musculature associated with the backbone and ribs. Still another portion of the somites, the *dermatome,* produces much of the deeper portions of the skin, the *dermis.*

The bones of the skull and face are derived directly from membranous tissue in the dermis of those regions beginning in the fifth and sixth weeks of gestation. The appendicular skeleton (the shoulder and pelvic girdles and their appendages) are preformed in cartilage. This cartilage is later broken down by special cells and bone salts are laid down in their place by still other cells. The limb buds arise from somatopleure and the skeletal elements appear to derive from this same embryonic tissue. The

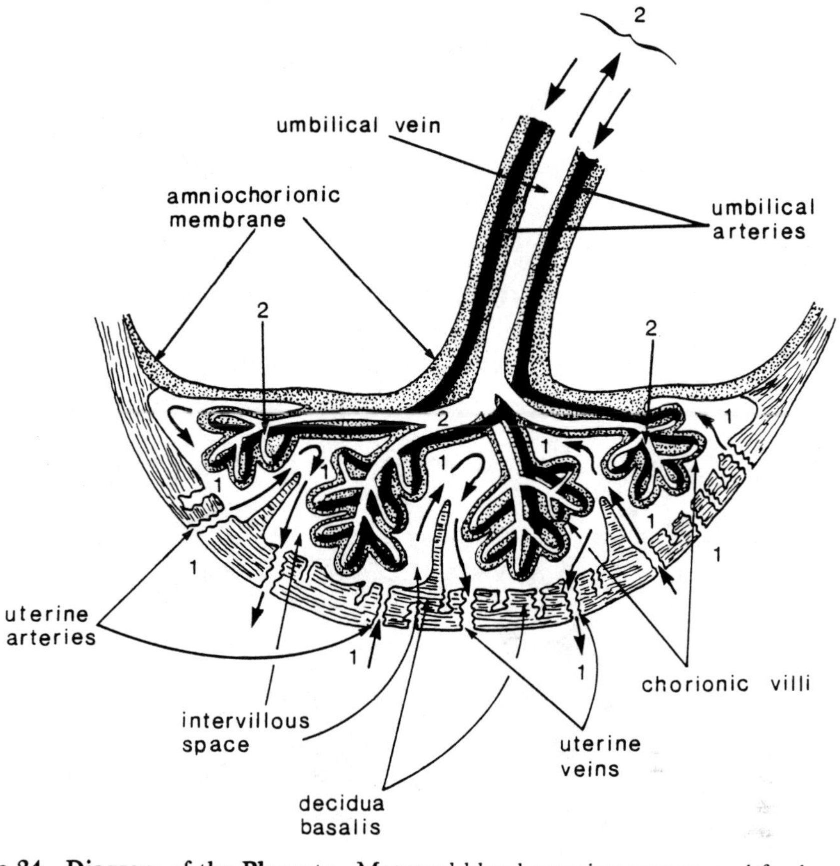

Figure 24. Diagram of the Placenta. Maternal blood carrying oxygen and food materials enters the intervillous spaces via numerous spirally-shaped uterine arteries (1). The blood is directed up against the underside of the "plate" formed by the amniochorionic membrane in intermittent spurts, bathing the chorionic villi and allowing the exchange of gases and other materials: CO_2 and waste products from the fetal to the maternal blood, and O_2 and nutrients from the maternal to the fetal blood. Large and intermediate sized arrows show the direction of the maternal (1) and fetal (2) blood flow, which are completely separate from one another. These molecules diffuse across the placental barrier, which consists of the trophoblast and underlying capillary endothelium of the chorionic villi. The placental barrier becomes much thinner with advancing pregnancy until it is as little as 0.002 mm thick (Arey 1965), allowing for greatly increased transfer rate in both directions. Black-colored vessels are outgoing fetal arteries and arterioles carrying spent, deoxygenated blood to the chorionic villi; white vessels are venules and veins carrying freshly oxygenated and food-laden blood from the villi to the fetus.

complex details of bone development are outside the scope of this work.

Further organogenesis occurs by development of the primordial structures already differentiated during this period and will not be elaborated further here. The viscera, including the entire digestive tract, the

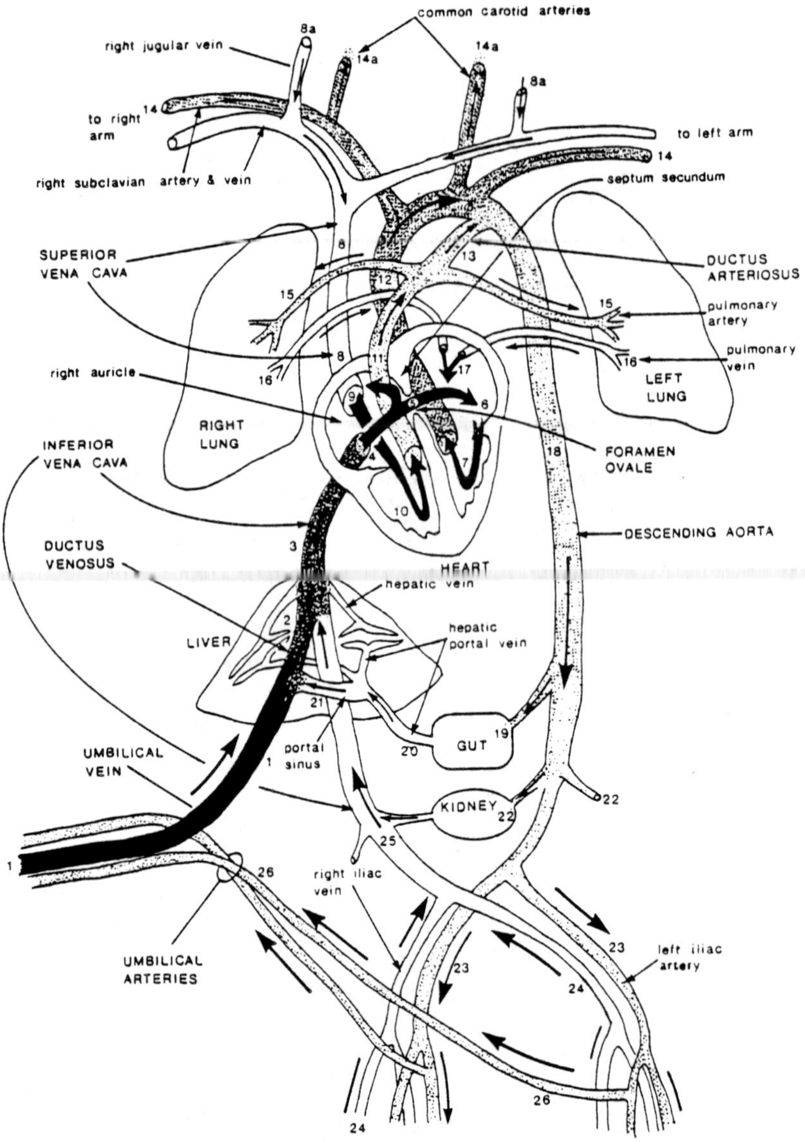

Figure 25. Fetal Circulation. The degree of oxygen saturation of the blood in this figure is indicated by the degree of shading: darker vessels carry more oxygenated blood, intermediate saturation is indicated by relative stippling, and white (non-shaded) vessels carry spent, deoxygenated blood. The dark arrows showing blood flow do not relate to oxygen saturation.

Freshly oxygenated blood is carried from the placenta by the large *umbilical vein* (1) through the liver via a temporary, embryonic structure, the *ductus venosus* (2) to the *inferior (posterior) vena cava* (3) with which it merges. The oxygenated blood from the placenta is mixed with deoxygenated blood from both the inferior vena cava and the *hepatic portal vein* (20) via the *portal sinus* (21). This mixed, partially oxygenated blood enters the *right auricle* via the *sinus venosus* (4), a common chamber into which both the inferior and superior venae cavae empty. This mixed blood streams across the right auricle and part of it is diverted back into the right auricle by the *septum secundum,* the wall which divides the right and left auricles. That portion of the blood diverted back into the right auricle then enters the *right* →

ventricle along with fully spent, deoxygenated blood from the *superior (anterior) vena cava* (10). However, the bulk of the blood from the inferior vena cava enters the left auricle through a small, temporary window (which closes at birth) called the *foramen ovale* (5). It is then passed into the *left ventricle* (6 and 7) along with the small amount of blood coming into the left auricle from the *pulmonary veins* (16). This moderately oxygenated blood from the left ventricle is then sent out through the *ascending aorta* or *aortic arch* (12) wherefrom it is distributed to: the right side of the anterior body via a trunk branching off from the aortic arch called the *brachiocephalic artery* (not labelled) and into the *right subclavian artery* (14) leading into the right arm and the *right common carotid artery* (14a) carrying blood to the head and brain; at the apex of the aortic arch the blood from the left ventricle is carried into the head region via the *right common carotid artery* and into the left arm through the *left subclavian artery* (14). The blood richest in oxygen content is thus shunted by the most direct route through the fetal heart and into the aortic arch, and thence into the developing brain with its high oxygen requirements. *Note that this blood is only partially oxygenated at best because of mixing with deoxygenated blood from the inferior vena cava (25), the hepatic portal vein (20) and spent blood coming into the right auricle from the superior vena cava draining the anterior body region (8)!* Blood leaving the right ventricle of the heart (10) contains significantly less oxygen than that from the left ventricle because it is diluted by spent blood from the superior vena cava (8 and 9). In order to prevent most of this blood from going out into the lungs (which are nonfunctional during fetal development) via the *pulmonary arteries* (15) and thence back into the left auricle where it would further dilute the blood going to the head, blood from the right ventricle is shunted past the lungs by another temporary fetal structure, the *ductus arteriosus* (13), which atrophies soon after birth. This blood is normally carried into the functional lungs where oxygen transfer occurs in the postnatal circulation; however, in the fetal system oxygenation occurs at the placenta, and the ductus arteriosus prevents too much dilution of the blood going to the head region during the fetal period. The blood leaving the right side of the heart (10 and 11) is largely deoxygenated, and to prevent its mingling with the blood from the left side of the heart, the ductus arteriosus joins the aortic arch at a point beyond that at which the oxygenated blood is sent to the anterior body region. The remainder of the partially oxygenated blood from the aortic arch goes into the *descending aorta* (18) and is distributed to the lower body region where oxygen requirements are less critical (19 to 23). Nearly-spent blood is carried from the fetus to the placenta via the *umbilical arteries* (26). Deoxygenated blood from the anterior body region is carried back to the superior vena cava (and thence to the heart) via the *jugular veins* (8a) from the head and neck, which joins the left and right *subclavian veins* to form the left and right *brachiocephalic veins* [not labelled]. The brachiocephalic veins then fuse to form the large superior vena cava (8).

This system for providing maximally oxygenated blood to the most critical tissues of the head is marginal at best. Any factor which disrupts or impairs the already barely adequate circulation can severely impact against the proper development of fetal tissues and organs, resulting in congenital malformations and/or impairment of growth and functioning. At birth, the ductus venosus, ductus arteriosus, foramen ovale, and the umbilical vasculature atrophy and disappear, except for remnants of the umbilical veins which persist in the adult and which connect the left hepatic portal vein with the *epigastric veins* of the systemic circulation. This remnant can play a role in the development of medical complications due to alcoholic portal hypertension (see Light 1985). In postnatal circulation, blood from the superior and inferior venae cavae enter the right auricle via a common chamber known as the *sinus venosus,* and since in adult circulation the foramen ovale has closed, this deoxygenated blood is transported from the right ventricle out through the *pulmonary trunk* (11) and into the lungs via the *pulmonary arteries* (15). The blood is oxygenated in the lungs and carbon dioxide is given off, and the freshly oxygenated blood is carried to the left auricle via the *pulmonary veins* (16 and 17). It then enters the left ventricle and is pumped out into the ascending aorta and to all parts of the body.

lungs, liver, pancreas, gall bladder and related structures all arise as simple outpockets of the gut. The details are not important to this discussion. The derivatives of the three major germ layers can be summarized (after Moore 1977):

ECTODERM:	Surface Ectoderm:	the skin and related structures (hair, nails, etc.), mammary glands, anterior lobe of pituitary gland, enamel of teeth, inner ear, lens of the eye.
	Neuroectoderm:	*neural tube:* brain and spinal cord, retina of the eye, pineal gland, posterior lobe of pituitary gland.
		neural crest cells: cranial nerves, peripheral nervous system, adrenal medulla, pigment cells.
MESODERM:	Paraxial Mesoderm:	muscles of trunk, skeleton except for the skull, dermis of the skin, connective tissue.
	Intermediate Mesoderm:	urogenital system and accessory structures.
	Lateral Plate Mesoderm:	connective tissue (mesenteries) of viscera and heart, blood and lymph cells, circulatory system, spleen, adrenal cortex.
	Head Mesoderm:	skull and bones of the face, dentine of teeth.
ENDODERM:		The viscera, lungs, bladder, lining of the trachea, bronchi, pharynx, and the thyroid and parathyroid glands, and tonsils.

By day 24 the first two pairs of branchial or gill arches appear (Figure 21), each enclosing a cartilaginous support and an aortic arch derived from the paired dorsal aortae. The first such arch or *mandibular process* (Figure 26A) will soon bifurcate on each side, giving rise to the *maxillary* and *mandibular processes.* The former will produce the upper jaw and the latter the lower jaw or mandible. In addition, portions of the first arch forms two of the bones of the middle ear, the *malleus* and the *incus*[66] The second or *hyoid arch* give rise to the third middle ear ossicle, the *stapes,*

[66] An example of ontogeny recapitulating phylogeny. This same branchial arch gave rise to the middle ear ossicles in the evolutionary transition from fish through amphibian and reptile to mammal.

and contributes to the formation of the *hyoid cartilage*. The remaining branchial arches, of which five will ultimately appear as transient structures in the human fetus, give rise to a variety of adult structures, notably the cartilages and their associated ligaments of the pharynx and larynx and certain muscles of the tongue and face. The gut endoderm lining the inner surface of the branchial arches gives rise to the thymus and parathyroid glands and portions of the thyroid gland, and also contributes to the middle ear architecture. The oropharyngeal membrane has also ruptured by day 24 forming the *stomodaeum*. The ectoderm of the mouth is now confluent with the endoderm of the pharynx.

Because facial abnormalities form so prominent a suite of characteristics of the fetal alcohol syndrome, the development of this region will be discussed in some detail. Five *facial primordia* or germinative regions are present early in the fourth gestational week (Figure 26A): a median, unpaired *frontonasal prominence*, paired *maxillary processes*, and paired *mandibular processes*. *Nasal placodes* are established by the end of the fourth week, each with a prominent horseshoe-shaped margin. The inner and outer borders of this horseshoelike structure are termed the *median* and *lateral nasal processes* or *prominences*, respectively (Figure 26B). A *nasal pit* develops in each of the nasal placodes and a cleft, the *nasolabial groove* connects each nasal pit with the stomodeum and separates each lateral nasal prominence from the adjacent maxillary process.

The bulk of facial development occurs during the fifth to eighth weeks. The several process and prominences just described represent local centers of mesenchymal[67] proliferation. As these regions develop, the furrows between them tend to smooth out. The lower jaw develops first by a fusion of the lower ends of the paired mandibular processes. The upper jaw develops somewhat later by the merging of the two median nasal prominences and the paired maxillary processes (Figure 26B-E). This merging of the upper jaw elements takes place during gestational weeks six and seven. The medial nasal prominences merge with each other to form an intermaxillary section lying between the two converging maxillary processes. This section gives rise to the *philtrum* or median, vertical furrow of the human upper lip, the associated gum region, and the primary palate. The lateral portion of the upper lip and jaw and the secondary palate are formed from the maxillary processes.

[67] *Mesenchyme* refers to rapidly proliferating, undifferentiated, embryonic tissue possessing a wide developmental potential, that is, it can become a variety of different tissue types. Once it starts to differentiate into specific cell types, however, this early wide potential becomes more and more restricted as to what can be formed.

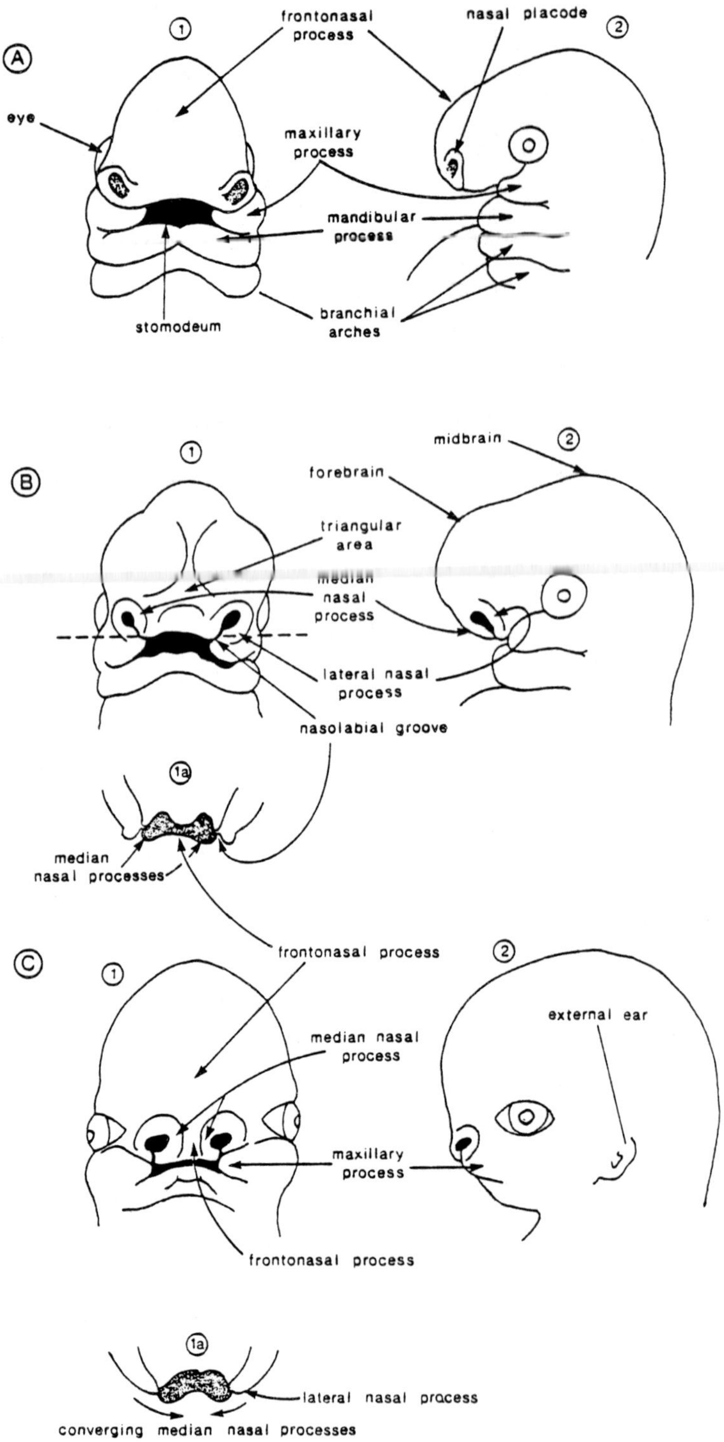

Figure 26. Human Facial Development. A. Embryo at about day 28. The first branchial arch has differentiated into the maxillary and mandibular processes. The nasal placode is already present (not labelled) and the eyes have begun to form on the sides of the →

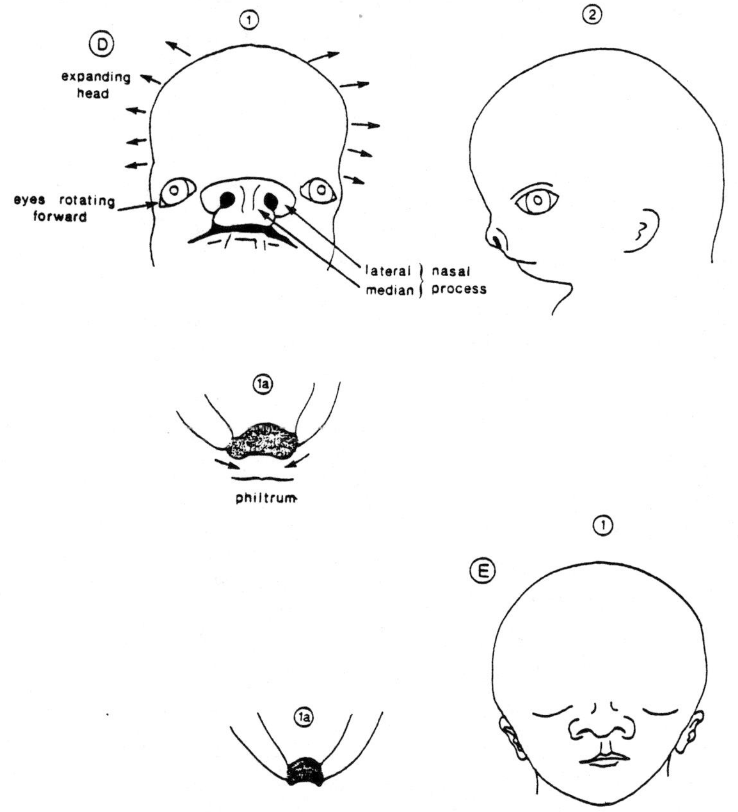

head. **B.** Five-week-old embryo. The median and lateral nasal processes (prominences) have developed around the nasal placodes; the nasal placodes themselves have developed into the forerunners of the nostrils, the nasal pits. Each nasal pit is connected to the stomodeum by a nasolabial groove. The median nasal processes and the lower portion of the frontonasal process are beginning to fuse into what will become the philtrum. The maxillary processes are converging, and together with the median nasal and lower part of the frontonasal processes will form the upper jaw. **C.** The face at about the end of the fifth week. The medial nasal prominences are merging with each other and with the maxillary processes. **D.** Facial development during the sixth week. The lower part of the nose and the upper lip have formed. The eyes have rotated forward as a consequence of the posterior expansion of the brain and skull (arrows). As the median nasal and maxillary processes continue to fuse with each other, the nasolabial grooves will become obliterated and the cells from these primordia will smooth out. Eventually, only the philtrum will remain as a remnant of these several processes. **E.** The face at about 14 weeks. 1 = frontal view of the face; 2 = left lateral view; 1a = dorsal view of section through upper jaw. After Arey 1965 and Moore 1977.

The facial abnormalities characteristic of FAS appear to result from hypoplasia or underdevelopment of the frontonasal process and its embryonic derivatives, in particular the median nasal processes and the triangular area. Deficiencies in the medial nasal processes result in a reduced or absent philtrum, and also permit the maxillary processes to converge more completely than they otherwise would, resulting in a long (high) upper lip (see Figure 15). The small nose results from inadequate development of the lower frontonasal and medial nasal processes. Eye malformations are common, and the shortened palpebral fissures reflect a primary growth deficiency. They remain widely spaced apart because of inadequate growth of the brain and posterior braincase. [After Sulik *et al.* 1981.]

The frontonasal process corresponds to the forehead region. The lower portion of the frontonasal process is known as the *triangular area* (Figure 26B). The triangular area will form the bridge and apex of the nose and the lateral nasal processes will give rise to the sides and flared *alae* or "wings" of the nostrils. The lateral nasal processes also merge with their respective maxillary processes. The nose is at first broad and flat and the nostrils are placed rather far apart. Later in fetal life the bridge will become elevated and the nostrils directed downward. The lower jaw is similarly underdeveloped, attaining its normal development after week 14. These facial changes are accompanied by rapid growth of the brain and expansion of the skull (Figure 26D). This growth, especially of the posterior skull region, causes the eyes, which had developed on the sides of the head (Figure 26B-C) to converge medially (Figure 26E) so that they come to face directly forward, thus permitting stereoscopic or binocular (three-dimensional) vision.

To summarize: during the first three weeks of development the fertilized egg undergoes cleavage to form a hollow blastocyst which becomes implanted in the uterine wall. The inner cell mass gives rise to the amnion and the epiblast and hypoblast layers are established. The transient primary yolk sac arises from extraembryonic mesoderm derived from the cytotrophoblast; this is soon replaced with secondary yolk sac formed from hypoblastic cells. The bilaminar (two-layered) embryo becomes trilaminar (three-layered) by ingression of intraembryonic mesoderm from the primitive groove and knot. Chorionic villi from the embryo invade the uterine endometrium, and together with the decidua basalis form the placenta. The placenta becomes highly vascularized in order to transport oxygen and nutrients to and waste substances from the embryo.

Although the terms *embryo* and *fetus* have been used interchangeably in the discussion thus far, strictly speaking, developmental weeks four through eight represent the *embryonic period* (Moore 1977). During this time, the embryo and extraembryonic membranes undergo complex folding maneuvers and the embryo is transformed from a flat, three-layered, to a cylindrical conformation. The amnion expands to completely obliterate the extraembryonic coelom and forms an external sheath around the umbilical cord. All the major tissues and organ systems arise from the three germ layers during this period and the external features and appendages begin to appear. Branchial arches arise and become transformed into their adult derivatives, including the upper and lower jaws and parts of the face. By the end of the second month of gestation nearly all of the major organs have formed and subsequent development involves essentially the growth and refinement of these structures.

The ninth week up through birth represents the *fetal period.* Body growth and weight gain are very rapid during this period, and the fetus has become distinctly human in appearance. The head constitutes nearly one half of the entire fetal length (crown to rump) at the beginning of week nine, but by week 12 the body length has more than doubled whereas the relative rate of head growth has slowed down considerably. The arms, which began as small limb buds during week four, have almost reached their normal length relative to the body at the end of week 12, although the legs are still somewhat reduced (having first appeared as limb buds a few days later than the arms). The external genitalia, which at week nine were similar, have become sexually differentiated by the twelfth week. And some reflex activity is also present by this time.

During the third month (weeks 13 to 16) fetal growth is extremely rapid, and the head to body ratio begins to approach that of the perinatal period. The axial and appendicular skeletons, which had already begun to form as cartilaginous precursors, begin to ossify and some of the cartilaginous elements are slowly replaced by bone during the third and subsequent months. The bones of the skull base are derived from cartilaginous masses in the head and branchial arches which later become ossified. The sides and roof of the skull, however, are formed directly as bone laid down by mesenchymal membranes without any cartilaginous forerunners. Complete ossification of the skeleton does not occur until much later in life; this is particularly true of the limb bones in which final ossification occurs at puberty when final body size is attained. During the third month the body gradually straightens out from its hunched-over embryonic shape and the posture becomes more upright. Nails, hair and tooth buds appear, the kidneys begin to function and swallowing motions become evident.

During the fourth and fifth months growth continues, the fluid-filled and as yet non-functional lungs are formed, and embryonic movements are now felt by the mother. Complex reflexes have appeared and the eyes are light sensitive. Because the respiratory system is still quite immature, 25-week-old fetuses usually die if born prematurely. A light, downy body hair, the *lanugo,* and a cheesy secretion from the fetal skin, the *vernix caseosa,* cover the body. The lanugo and vernix appear to protect the fetus from abrasions and skin hardening.

During the sixth month abundant scalp hair, eyebrows and eyelashes develop. The skin has become well vascularized and the fetus may drink amniotic fluid and engage in thumb-sucking. The viscera are still largely nonfunctional and temperature regulation and rhythmic breathing are usually not yet possible, and fetuses prematurely born at this stage rarely survive.

Although the mortality rate is high for fetuses born during the seventh month, survival is now possible because the lungs and their blood supply are adequate to allow for gas exchange. The central nervous system is also mature enough to control rhythmic breathing and maintain body temperature.

The eighth and ninth months constitute a finishing stage. The rapid growth of earlier periods slows down considerably as the fetus comes to fill the entire amniotic space. The placenta also becomes fibrous and less functional about this time. Antibodies from the maternal blood provide immunity from disease for the first several months of postnatal life. About one third of all premature infants are also small for their gestational age, and this often results from placental insufficiency. Such *intrauterine growth retardation* as opposed to small weight and size due to shortened gestation is also caused by genetic and environmental factors such as prenatal exposure to drugs and other teratogenic agents.

Birth usually occurs at about 266 days or 38 weeks following fertilization and most babies are born within ten to 15 days before or after this time. Fetal liver enzymes, particularly the microsomal enzymes (see Light 1985), exhibit low activity at this time, at least in most cases. Prior to birth unconjugated bilirubin deriving from red blood cell breakdown (see Light 1985) in the fetus is readily transported across the placenta from the fetal to the maternal circulation, whereupon it is then detoxified by the maternal liver (Pritchard and MacDonald 1976). Unconjugated bilirubin cannot be excreted since it is not water-soluble. The mature liver normally conjugates bilirubin with glucuronic acid to form a water-soluable glucuronide which can be eliminated via the bile into the feces, or via the kidneys when plasma levels become elevated. *Glucuronyl transferase,* the enzyme which catalyzes this conjugation reaction, is associated with the hepatic microsomal enzyme system. Premature infants especially are deficient in glucuronyl transferase activity, and they often develop *hyperbilirubinemia* or elevated plasma levels of bilirubin which can result in a toxic and dangerous jaundice.

Uridine diphosphate glucuronic acid (UDP-glucuronic acid) is formed from *UDP-glucose* by the enzyme *UDP-glucose dehydrogenase* in a reaction involving the reduction of NAD^+ to NADH. UDP-glucuronic acid is then conjugated with a variety of substrates by UDP-glucuronyl transferase to form a *glucuronide,* which being water soluble, is readily excreted

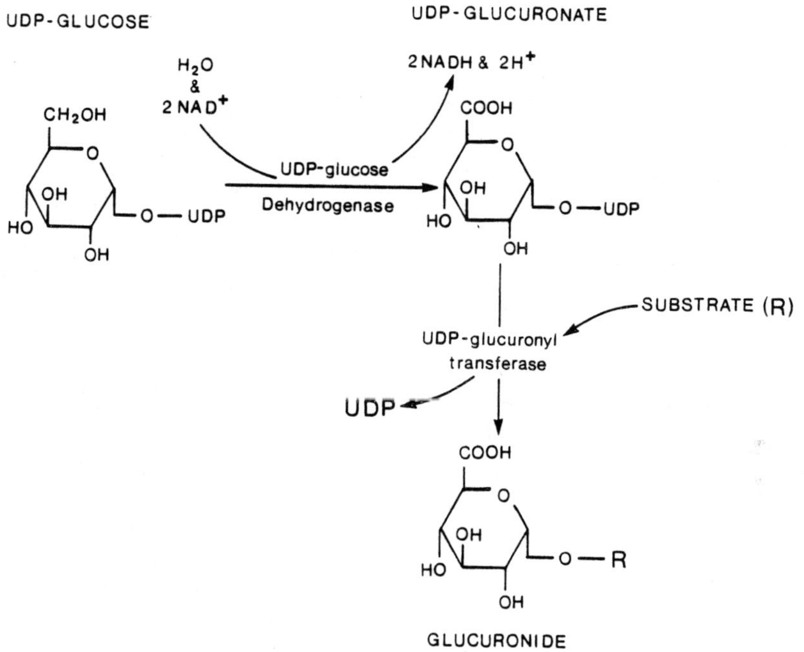

Figure 27. Glucuronide Formation. UDP-glucuronic acid is formed from UDP-glucose in a reaction catalyzed by UDP-glucose dehydrogenase in which NAD^+ is reduced to NADH. UDP-glucuronate is then conjugated with a variety of substrates by UDP-glucuronyl transferase to form a glucuronide, which is then excreted in the feces or urine.

by the feces or urine (see Figure 27). Unconjugated bilirubin is carried in the blood attached to binding sites on plasma albumin. Normally it is taken up by the liver cells and conjugated into glucuronide. When plasma bilirubin levels exceed the carrying capacity of the plasma albumin or when bilirubin is competitively excluded from the albumin binding sites by other substrates, the free, unconjugated and highly lipid-soluble bilirubin readily crosses the blood-brain barrier and is taken up by neural membranes.

When *physiological jaundice* occurs in the newborn baby due to the lack of microsomal enzyme activity, it usually increases for three or four days up to levels of 10 mg per 100 ml, thereafter falling rapidly as liver enzymes come up to effective activity. The jaundice is often more prolonged and more intense in premature infants.[68] Bilirubin toxicity is aggravated by the presence of drugs such as sulfonamides commonly

[68]Seriously jaundiced newborns, particularly those of low weight, although they may otherwise be normal, are commonly treated by phototherapy with simulated sunlight. Light penetrates the infant's skin and photooxidizes bilirubin. It also promotes excretion of unconjugated bilirubin by the liver by an unknown mechanism.

given to pregnant women with urinary tract infections, and salicylates such as aspirin. These drugs compete with unconjugated bilirubin for the albumin binding sites, and plasma levels of free bilirubin are thus elevated. Hypoxia and acidosis likewise reduce the bound fraction of unconjugated bilirubin and also contribute to bilirubin toxicity.

Kernicterus is a common complication of uncompensated hyperbilirubinemia among newborn infants and this complication is more frequent among premature babies. Severe and widespread lesions develop in the cerebral grey matter and basal ganglia of the brain following birth in this disorder. These lesions result from the lipid-solubility of free unconjugated bilirubin which becomes deposited in these degenerative sites, typically producing a yellowish color in the affected areas. Those infants which survive such a neonatal kernicterus may suffer serious and global neurological effects involving regional neural degeneration and ensuing hyperdevelopment of the glial cells.

The presence of drugs such as barbiturates in the fetal blood induce the microsomal liver enzymes into greater activity—this is particularly true of cytochrome P-450 and UDP-glucuronyl transferase. Babies born to drug-taking women therefore commonly exhibit "revved-up livers" and they are able to readily conjugate bilirubin as well as metabolize a variety of drugs at birth. Because of the ability of barbiturates to induce UDP-glucuronyl transferase, they are commonly administered as a therapeutic measure against neonatal hyperbilirubinemia.

Ethanol is not specifically linked to neonatal hyperbilirubinemia or the development of kernicterus. Although probably a substrate for glucuronyl transferase, it is a much weaker competitor for this enzyme system than are the secondary and tertiary alcohols.[69] However, alcohol is known to inhibit the synthesis of UDP-glucuronic acid from UDP-glucose by altering the liver redox state in favor of a higher NADH: NAD^+ ratio (Lieber 1983).[70] Alcohol abuse is often associated with polydrug abuse, particularly among women, and they frequently consume barbiturates and benzodiazepines in addition to alcohol. The maternal consumption of barbiturates late in the course of pregnancy will enhance the neonate's ability to conjugate bilirubin and thus clear it from the blood. Unlike the barbiturates, both ethanol and benzodiazepines such as Valium® are sequestered into the mammary glands of

[69] This appears to be a function of the higher lipid-water partition coefficient of the latter alcohols.

[70] See Light 1985. NAD^+ is reduced to NADH in the oxidation of ethanol to acetaldehyde and of acetaldehyde to acetate. The consequent buildup of reducing equivalents is responsible for most of the biochemical malfunctions that result from alcohol abuse.

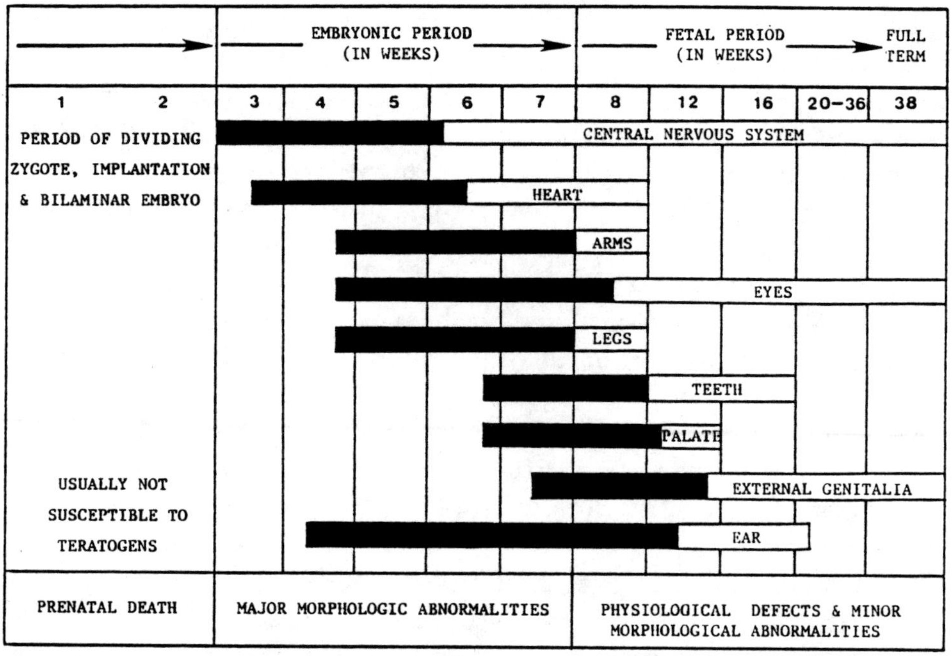

Figure 28. Teratogens and the Critical Periods of Human Development. Solid black bars denote periods of high sensitivity to the actions of teratogens; white bars indicate periods of less susceptibility. The bottom row of boxes specify the main developmental problems encountered during the periods indicated. After figures by Moore 1973 and Harbison 1980. Exposure to teratogens in the pre-implantation period is associated with lethality, but not with gross structural and functional malformations. The latter occur mainly during the period of organogenesis, from about 18 through 60 days following conception. Thereafter, the fetus is increasingly resistant to gross structural malformations, but is still vulnerable to deficiencies in growth and maturation, which can result in intrauterine growth retardation and functional disturbances. The full fetal alcohol syndrome appears to be the result of exposure throughout prenatal development (Chernoff 1980).

lactating mothers and are consumed by the nursing infant in the mother's milk. Benzodiazepines compete directly with bilirubin for glucuronyl transferase and are conjugated with glucuronic acid. Ethanol, as just noted, suppresses the synthesis of glucuronic acid by reducing and thus tying up all the available NAD^+. Both alcohol and the benzodiazepines could therefore contribute to the development of hyperbilirubinemia in newborn infants and perhaps contribute to the development of kernicterus. Such an interaction has not been demonstrated, however.

The most important single factor in any drug-induced teratogenesis is the gestational age of the embryo or fetus. During the first two weeks of human development, the embryo is relatively non-susceptible to teratogenic action. A toxic agent either damages all of the predifferentiating embryo and causes its death, or it injures only a few as yet undifferentiated cells which are readily replaced so that the embryo can recover without developmental abnormalities (Moore 1977). Human organogenesis begins on about day 21 or the first somite stage and it continues through the third month. Toxic insults sustained during this period are likely to result in major morphological abnormalities, particularly to the central nervous system. The second trimester reflects the period of finer morphological and biochemical differentiation. The third trimester is involved primarily with growth and physiological development. Exposure to toxic agents during these later periods of fetal development is more likely to cause minor to moderate functional disturbances rather than gross structural malformations. The fetus becomes increasingly resistant to teratogenesis with advancing gestational age, and growth and functional retardation are the likely results of environmental insult during these later stages. [See Figure 28.]

Drugs and other toxic agents also cross the placental barrier at differing rates during development. Lipid soluble agents readily cross the placenta into the fetal circulation during the early stages of placental development. As the placenta matures, the transfer rate drops markedly. The mature placenta is also an important site of drug and other xenobiotic biotransformation. This capacity on the part of the placenta to biotransform drugs becomes more pronounced with increasing gestational age. These biotransformation reactions include: oxidation, reduction, hydroxylation, and conjugation (Harbison and Evans 1977); placental biotransformation may approach the rates seen in adult hepatic tissue. Placental biotransformation undoubtedly provides a significant buffer against the introduction of many foreign molecules into the fetal circulation. As we have seen, it may prevent the transfer of acetaldehyde consequent to ethanol oxidation into the fetal tissues (see above). Late in the course of pregnancy, placental deterioration and death again permits a rapid rate of transport of lipophilic agents from the maternal into the fetal compartments.

The presence of biotransforming enzymes in the placenta present an increased risk to the fetus of drug toxicity as well as a protecting buffer. Biotransformation typically converts a relatively non-toxic and lipophilic compound into a polar, water-soluble, and often more reactive, toxic substance (see Light 1985 for a more detailed discussion). The activity of these biotransforming enzymes tend to increase the concentrations of polar metabolites in the fetal circulation, and excretion of these

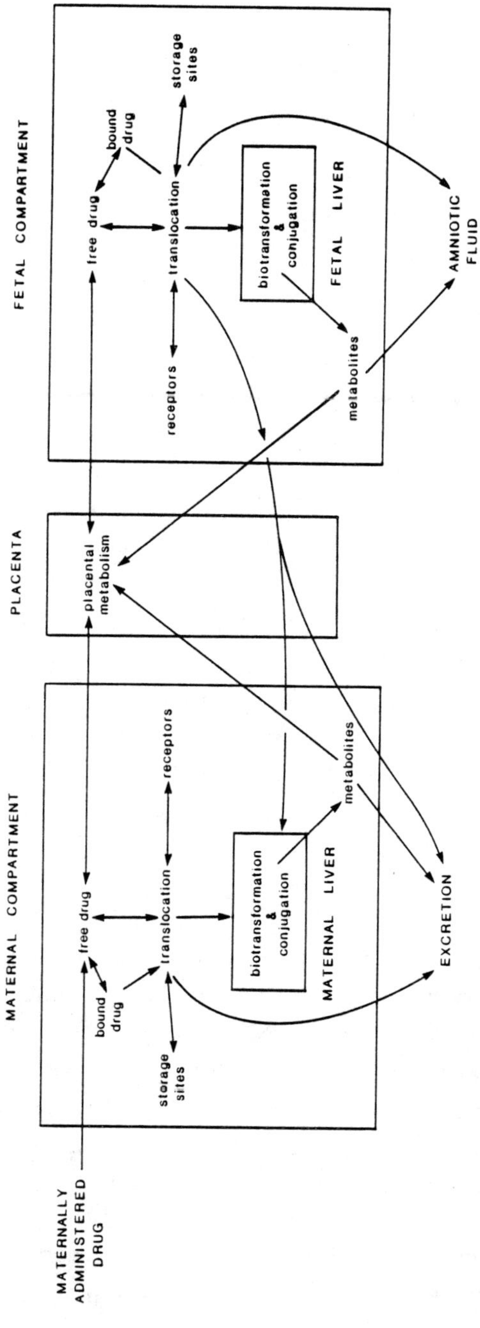

Figure 29. Drug Disposition in the Maternal-Placental-Fetal Compartments. Partly after Harbison and Evans 1977.

lipophobic compounds from the fetal compartment across the placenta would be restricted. Clearance from the fetal compartment would be further impaired by the presence of these same metabolites in the maternal circulation. Thus, competitive inhibition of drug clearance from maternal circulation by other drugs would result in elevated levels of the drug in both the maternal and fetal compartments. Fetal drug and metabolite concentrations tend to parallel maternal plasma concentrations.

Although fetal liver microsomal enzymes typically exhibit much lower activity levels than are found later in life, these enzymes are capable of being induced *in utero* by challenges resulting from maternal exposure to drugs and other xenobiotics. The case with respect to barbiturates has already been described. However, there appears to be wide variation in the ability of fetal liver enzymes to metabolize different types of drugs. Because the fetal liver is relatively larger than the adult liver (relative to body size), the fetus in some circumstances may be able to metabolize certain drugs much more rapidly than the mother can (Harbison and Evans 1977). Because the metabolites of these drugs would presumably be more polar than their lipophilic precursors, they would tend not to be transported across the placental barrier for excretion by the maternal compartment. As a result they would tend to accumulate within the fetal tissues where, fetal tissues being much more susceptible to drug-induced damage, they have the potential for causing major damage. The dynamics of drug distribution and metabolism between the maternal, placental, and fetal compartments is summarized in Figure 29.

Alcohol probably causes fetal damage by means of: (1) direct cytotoxic insult to the fetal tissues, (2) direct cytotoxic damage to fetal tissues by one or more metabolites such as acetaldehyde, (3) impairment of normal cell division and migration during early embryonic life, and (4) indirect damage to fetal tissues due to hypoxia, acidosis, and other altered metabolic states in both the maternal and fetal compartments. Although acetaldehyde has not yet been demonstrated in human fetal tissues in response to maternal alcohol intake, it is accepted by nearly all investigators that it probably does cross the placental barrier and is very likely responsible for many of the gross defects associated with fetal alcohol syndrome. It may be especially important as a cause of neurological defects (Pratt 1980).

It is thought that acetaldehyde can accumulate in fetal tissues by being generated from ethanol metabolism in the maternal liver. And since alcohol, like the barbiturates, induces fetal liver microsomal activity and appears also to be able to induce greater activity of alcohol dehydrogenase in fetal livers, at least in experimental animals (Rosett 1980), fetal acetaldehyde probably also derives from the oxidation of ethanol within the fetal liver. As previously noted, all or a significant portion of the maternally derived acetaldehyde may be oxidized by the placental tissues before it can cross over into the fetal compartment. Other factors that may act to reduce the fetal load of acetaldehyde include: (1) local oxidation of acetaldehyde in the maternal mitochondria, (2) oxidation by the maternal red blood cells during circulation from the maternal liver to the uterine artery, (3) oxidation by fetal red blood cells during passage from the placenta to the fetal tissues especially the brain, and (4) oxidation at the fetal blood-brain barrier (Pratt 1980).[71] On the other hand, acetaldehyde-induced disruption of both maternal and fetal mitochondrial membranes would reduce the oxidation of this substance and permit its escape into the circulation of both compartments.[72] Should acetaldehyde levels reach sufficient concentrations in the maternal circulation—not an improbable event in an alcoholic woman—all of the mechanisms inhibiting its transfer across the placental barrier could be overcome and the fetus exposed to toxic levels of this substance.

Although blood acetaldehyde levels are hundreds or even thousands of times less than blood alcohol concentrations, even in cases of severe intoxication (Wartburg 1980; Pratt 1980; Mukherjee and Hodgen 1982), its toxicity is much higher. Consequently, it can produce greater toxic effects than alcohol itself. The upper limits of blood alcohol concentration during even severe intoxication rarely exceed 100 mmoles/liter (about 460 mg/100 ml); levels greater than this are needed to impair the growth of cultured human lymphocytes (data in this paragraph are from Pratt 1980). Conversely, blood acetaldehyde concentrations of 40 mmoles/liter (about 0.2 mg/100 ml) will affect lymphocyte growth—a level commonly attained during severe intoxication. However, blood alcohol concentrations of 65 mmoles per liter (about 300 mg/

[71]Wartburg (1980) reported the existence of a previously unrecognized acetaldehyde oxidation mechanism in the form of aldehyde dehydrogenase within the membranes of red blood cells. This may represent a significant device for clearing acetaldehyde from the blood. In this regard, five different isozymes of aldehyde dehydrogenase are known from human liver and kidney tissues, each with varying levels of activity which are correlated with racial types and relative degrees of "flushing" due to acetaldehyde buildup. Electrophoretically different isozymes of aldehyde dehydrogenase are also reported from erythrocytes. [See Light 1985 for a discussion of general alcohol metabolism.]

[72]The oxidation of acetaldehyde into acetate takes place primarily in the liver mitochondria. [See Light 1985 for a discussion of this.]

100 ml) will adversely affect the growth of cultured cells in rat embryos; such a blood alcohol level is very commonly seen among alcoholics during intoxication. Both alcohol and acetaldehyde thus appear to be potentially toxic to embryonic tissue, and both probably play a major role in causing the congenital defects associated with fetal alcohol syndrome.

The abnormal migration of neural and glial cells onto the surface of the developing brain in humans and animal models known as *leptomeningeal neuroglial heterotopia* is a well-documented effect of repeated ethanol challenges to the fetus. The neural tube (Figure 20E-F) is originally a single layer of columnar cells. The lateral walls of this tube soon thicken and become pseudostratified into a columnar neuroepithelium (Figure 30) in which all the cells are anchored on a basement membrane bordering the neural canal. By the sixth gestational week the neural wall is bounded on the outer and inner surfaces by an *external* and *internal limiting membrane*, respectively. Three distinct layers are evident in the neural wall: (1) an inner (next to the neural canal) *ventricular zone* or *ependymal layer* which gives rise to all neural and glial cells and where the cell bases abut upon the internal limiting membrane; (2) an *intermediate zone* or *mantle layer* containing immature *neuroblasts,* destined to become neurons, which are derived from the ependymal layer; and (3) an outer *marginal layer* composed of the peripheral tips of the ependymal neuroepithelial cells. The neuroblasts of the mantle layer are generated by rapidly dividing cells of the ependymal layer. As these cells develop processes and mature into neurons they lose forever their ability to undergo mitosis and divide. All mitosis among the neuroblasts ceases before the end of the first postnatal year and the total number of neurons in the nervous system is fixed from that point on. The mantle layer will give rise to the future grey matter of the central nervous system. Nerve fibers grow into the marginal layer, which will give rise to the white matter of the CNS.

Most mitosis actually occurs within the ependymal layer. Even the dividing neuroblasts of the marginal layer round up and actually come to lie temporarily within the outer portion of the ependymal layer. After most neuroblast formation has taken place, mitotic activity in the ependymal layer gives rise to *spongioblasts* or *glioblasts* which migrate from the ependymal layer into the mantle and marginal layers where they differentiate into the various glial cells of the CNS—the astrocytes and oligodendrocytes.[73] Certain small neuroglial cells known as *microglial cells*

[73] See Light 1986a for a discussion of the nervous system. See also below, Appendix 2.

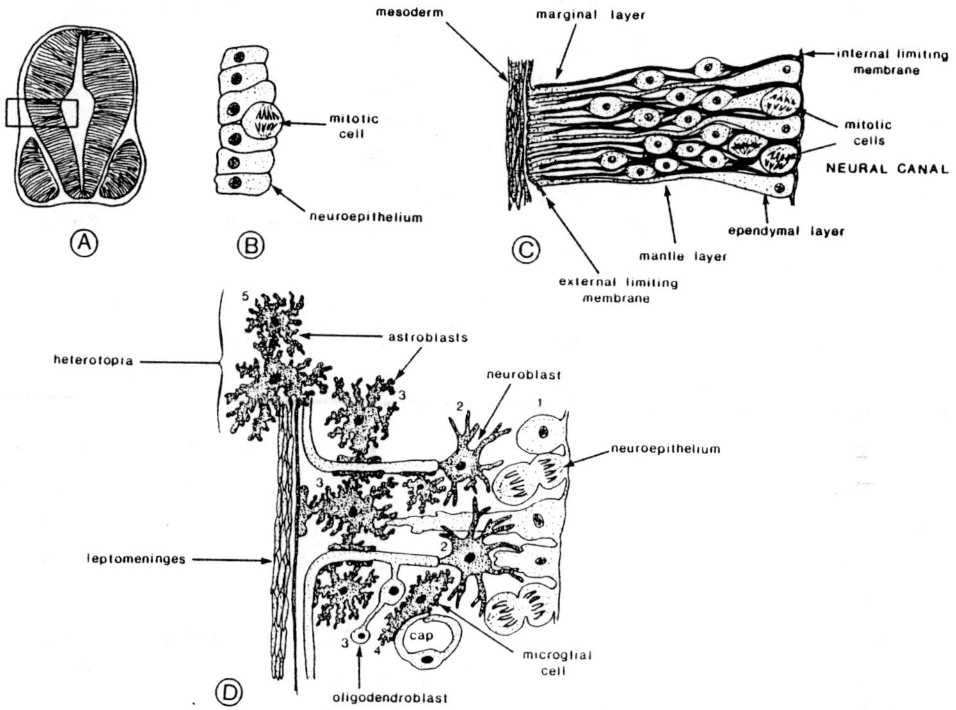

Figure 30. Differentiation of Neural Wall and Development of Leptomeningeal Heterotopia. A. Transverse section through neural tube—that illustrated here is at the level of the spinal cord. The rectangle outlines the region shown in the detail sections B to D. **B.** Single layer of columnar cells seen in the early, undifferentiated stage of neuroepithelial development. **C.** Later stage (about five to six weeks), showing pseudostratified neural wall, exhibiting the inner ependymal layer of actively mitotic (dividing) cells adjacent to the neural canal, the intermediate mantle layer, and the outermost marginal layer. Ependymal cells give rise first to neuroblasts, which themselves undergo multiple divisions and which migrate into the mantle layer and differentiate into neurons. Axons sprouting from the neuroblasts penetrate into the marginal layer. The ependymal cells secondarily give rise to spongioblasts (glioblasts) which migrate into the mantle and marginal layers. The spongioblasts will differentiate into astroblasts and oligodendroblasts—neuroglial cells which give rise to the supporting and nutritive astrocytes and the myelin sheath forming oligodendrocytes, respectively (see Light 1986a). **D.** Neural cell wall at a later stage of differentiation. The ependymal neuroepithelium (1) gives rise to the neuroblasts (2) which migrate into the mantle layer and differentiate into neurons. Neuroglial cells likewise arise from the ependymal layer and migrate into the mantle and marginal layers, where they differentiate into astroblasts and oligodendroblasts (3). Microglial cells (4) arise from the mesoderm lying outside the neural wall next to the external limiting membrane; these migrate inwardly into the marginal and mantle layers together with blood vessels derived from the same mesoderm. The leptomeninges (the pia mater and arachnoid) are likewise derived from this same outlying mesoderm. Under normal developmental circumstances, the migrating glial cells do not advance beyond the external limiting membrane. Heterotopia refers to the abnormal migration of neuroglial cells during certain developmental disorders; it is always associated with gross neurological impairment and mental retardation. Leptomeningeal neuroglial heterotopia, in which the neuroglial cells undergo excessive proliferation and push beyond the boundary of the neural wall and invade the leptomeningeal region (5), occurs in severe cases of fetal alcohol syndrome in both humans and animal models. Cap = crossection of a capillary.

differentiate from the mesenchyme (mesoderm) surrounding the neural tube and enter the CNS with the developing blood vessels. Differential proliferation and specialization of the neuroepithelial cells produce the thick walls and thinner roof and floor of the developing brain and all structures derived therefrom, with the exception of certain specialized organs like the anterior pituitary which derives from the roof of the pharynx. The *meninges*—three thin membranes which line the entire CNS—also appear to be derived from adjacent mesoderm, at least in humans.

Several studies have demonstrated a biphasic effect of ethanol upon the growth of different cells lines in culture (Syapin and Noble 1979). In extremely high doses—well in excess of 150 mM (about 690 mg/100 ml!), or more than twice the lethal dose to most tolerant alcohol addicts—ethanol inhibits cell growth and may cause irreversible damage to the line. However, much lower concentrations, ranging from 3.5 to 86 mM (about 16 to 395 mg/100 ml), stimulate mitosis and migration of a variety of embryonic chick and mammalian cell types. And this effect appears to be most pronounced during periods of otherwise rapid growth and differentiation. This is the same range of ethanol doses known to produce the abnormal glial cell migrations in fetal brains. Glial cell division and migration greatly exceeds normal rates, and penetration beyond the marginal layer of the brain into the leptomeningeal layers is the result. Fetal alcoholic heterotopia may therefore be related to the stimulatory effect that high, but sublethal doses of ethanol have upon embryonic cells *in vitro*. One study in which alcoholic leptomeningeal heterotopia was induced in an animal model reported a prevalence of mitotic activity in the neuroepithelium (Sulik *et al.* 1981). The mechanism underlying this response is not known. There is no evidence that acetaldehyde plays any role in this phenomenon.

The characteristic facial abnormalities of FAS (see Figures 15 and 16) may be interpreted as a general underdevelopment of the several facial primordia, in particular the embryonic derivatives of the frontonasal process (see Figure 26): the triangular area and the medial nasal processes (Sulik *et al.* 1981). The philtrum is normally formed by the fusion of the medial nasal processes (Figure 26C-D); the adequate development of the medial nasal processes also prevents the two maxillary process from converging completely. Inadequate development of the medial nasal processes appears to be associated with a reduced or absent philtrum, and because the maxillary processes are not prevented from converging together completely at the midline as normally occurs, a long, high upper lip characteristic of FAS commonly results (Figures 15 and 16). Inadequate development of the frontonasal process and the medial nasal processes produces a small nose with a very low bridge, and the forehead is also frequently narrow and underdeveloped. The entire midfacial region and lower jaw are typically underdeveloped, reflecting growth retardation of the maxillary and mandibular processes.

Shortened palpebral fissures commonly seen in FAS reflect a primary growth deficiency. Other eye malformations are also seen in FAS, including *microphthalmia* or smaller than normal eyes. The brain is typically very small and often exhibits blebs of abnormal glial tissue on its outer surface (leptomeningeal neuroglial heterotopia). The failure of the brain and the posterior braincase to expand as it normally does during development is often reflected by the failure of the eyes to move as far medially or forward on the face as they normally would, so that they remain spaced widely apart. All of these features have been reproduced in animal models (Sulik *et al.* 1981).

The wide variability in the effects of maternal drinking upon the fetus is due to a number of variables, of which perhaps the most critical is the gestational age of the embryo or fetus at which exposure occurs. The result of severe ethanol or other drug toxicity during the first two or three weeks of gestation is either death or resorption of the embryo; if the damage is less severe, the embryonic cells are still plastic enough that the effects may be overcome, leaving little in the way of obvious congenital malformations. Toxic injury during gestational weeks three to about eight or nine, the time of major organogenesis, often cause gross morphological deformities. In the case of FAS these typically involve characteristic abnormalities of the face, head and brain, and there may also be structural malformities of the heart and pericardial region. The brain is susceptible to damage at any stage during which nervous tissue is differentiating or neuronal and glial cells are migrating. These processes continue throughout fetal life and the first year following birth. During the third trimester the primary effects of teratogens including alcohol, and presumably also its metabolites, involve minor morphological defects, physiological deficits and malfunctions, growth retardation and failure to thrive. The late prenatal growth deficits due to FAS are usually not adequately compensated for by postnatal growth. These effects are summarized in Figure 28.

Maternal drinking patterns also play an important role in the genesis of fetal alcohol features. Chronic maternal drinking results in continuous high blood alcohol and acetaldehyde levels in the maternal, and one presumes, also in the fetal compartments. The insult is experienced throughout embryonic and fetal development, and continuous maternal drinking probably accounts for the most severe morphological and functional impairments seen in FAS babies. On the other hand, even one or two episodes of heavy drinking are capable of causing serious disruption of the fetal circulation because of total collapse of the placental blood vessels for periods of an hour or more, at least in monkeys (Mukherjee and Hodgen 1982; see also above).

Because fetal circulation under even the best of circumstances provides only marginal oxygenation to the developing brain (Figure 25), such a collapse could be expected to have potentially very serious consequences for the developing CNS. Alcoholics are characterized by higher blood acetaldehyde levels in response to alcohol intake than are nonalcoholics. This is due partly to the induction of alcohol metabolizing enzymes, resulting in more rapid conversion of ethanol to acetaldehyde, as well as to the impairment of acetaldehyde oxidation because of mitochondrial disruption caused by long-term alcohol abuse. It appears likely, therefore, that maternal plasma acetaldehyde levels may reach such proportions that spillover through the placental barrier into the fetal circulation may occur of sufficient intensity to overcome the various checks and barriers and reach the developing brain (Pratt 1980). Severe toxic injury to these vulnerable tissues from this metabolite even in very low concentrations is highly likely.

The resistance to toxic injury of different fetuses is also highly individual. Liver enzyme activity is also highly idiosyncratic as are the susceptibilities of these enzymes to induction by drugs and other xenobiotics. The specific drug-taking behavior of the mother is very relevant to this variable, and the maternal consumption of drugs such as barbiturates will tend to induce microsomal enzyme activity (see Light 1985) within the fetus, resulting in a buildup of toxic metabolites from a variety of precursors. Elevated cytochrome P-450 activity in the fetal liver could contribute to greater acetaldehyde buildup in the fetal circulation, enhancing the toxicity of that substance. Cigarette addiction, so prevalent among alcoholics, almost certainly exacerbates the growth retardation seen in fetal alcohol babies, and contributes to the smaller sizes and lower body weights so common among these infants. A major component of cigarette smoke is carbon monoxide, which binds irreversibly with haemoglobin and significantly impairs the ability of the red blood cells to carry oxygen. The resulting anoxia in the maternal compartment can only produce hypoxia within the fetus and add to the impact upon the developing child.

The medical consequences of chronic alcoholism to the mother also play an important role in the genesis of FAS. Hypoxia, acidosis, hypoglycemia, vitamin and mineral insufficiency, and altered amino acid metabolism due to the metabolic effects of alcohol insult in the mother can have serious negative consequences for the developing child, as would any degree of maternal liver failure and the toxic byproducts deriving therefrom. It is clear that there is *no safe level* of alcohol consumption for pregnant women! Quite apart from the general non-compliance of many alcoholic women with obstetrical advice about eating, drinking, smoking, and other drug-taking behavior, including "recreational," medically prescribed, and over-the-counter medications, a very real hazard relative to maternal alcohol consumption is that many women do not even know they are pregnant until significant alcohol-induced damage may already have taken place.

APPENDIX I

THE GENETIC information is carried within the DNA molecules coded in the sequence of the nitrogenous bases. Any sequence of the four base pairs is possible: AT, TA, CG, GC. Since the 46 chromosomes in humans contain an estimated ten billion base pairs, the possible sequential combinations are for all practical purposes without limit. In eukaryotes DNA is carried in the chromosomes, which also consist of proteins known as *histones*. In ordinary cell division or *mitosis* the DNA in each chromosome replicates itself by separating down the middle of the double strand in response to DNA polymerase (see above, Figure 2). Each of the original strands then provides, a template from which complementary strands are formed. Each complementary strand then moves away from the original template and serves as its own template from which complementary strands identical to the original are formed, resulting in two identical double-helices of DNA. In eukaryotes this process is accompanied by an exact twinning of each chromosome, resulting in the formation of two identical daughter *chromatids* joined together at a common point called the *centrosome* or *kinetochore.*

As mitosis proceeds, the replicated chromosomes line up in a single line in the middle of the cells (the *equatorial plane*). Each kinetochore then divides separating each of the chromatid pairs, which are then drawn toward opposite sides of the dividing cell by a complex system of *spindle fibers* attached to two bodies known as *centrioles.* When each chromatid pair separates and begin to move away from each other they are once again individual chromosomes. As they move apart the cytoplasm in the middle of the cell along the equatorial plane begins to constrict, ultimately separating the original cell into two daughter cells. Each daughter cell receives an exact duplicate of the original set of chromosomes in the original, undivided cell. This ensure that each daughter cell is genetically identical to the original cell.

The problems faced by developing gametes is somewhat different.

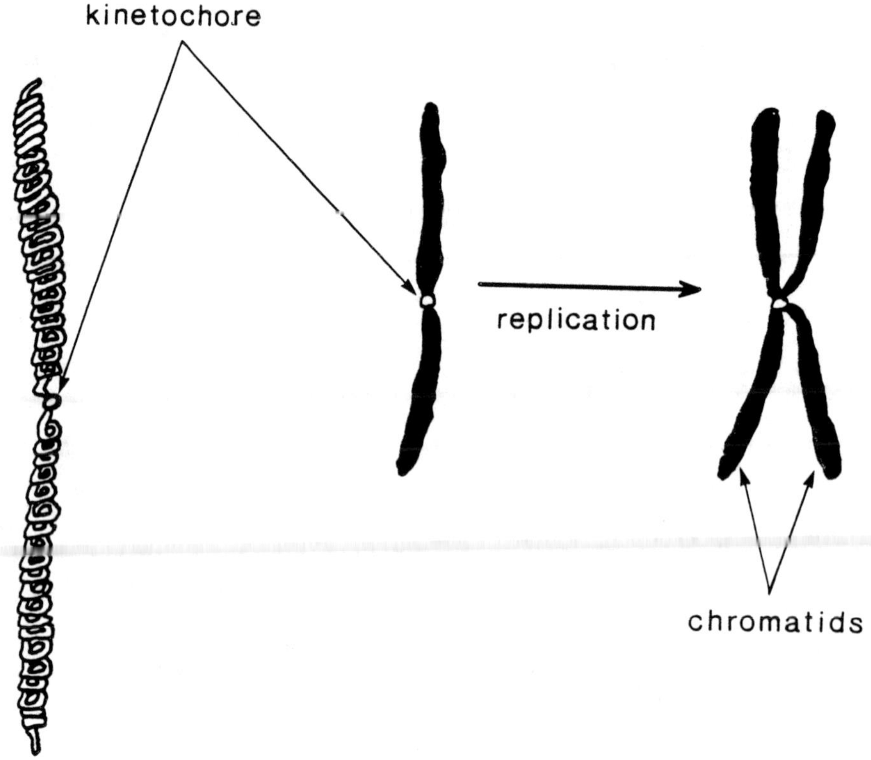

Because the adult human has 46 chromosomes (22 autosomes and two sex chromosomes)—known as the *diploid* number—each maturing germ cell must divest itself of exactly one-half of its diploid complement of chromosomes so that it has the proper *haploid* number. When the haploid egg and fertilizing spermatozoon come together, the resulting fusion of chromosomes from each again produces a diploid cell—now known as the *zygote.* The zygote then begins to undergo a great many mitotic divisions to eventually grow into an adult organism.

The process whereby developing gametes reduce their number of chromosomes is called *meiosis.* Meiosis is in many ways similar to mitosis and has evolved from it. But whereas mitosis occurs in one stage, meiosis requires two stages involving two successive divisions which results in four nuclei, each containing a haploid number of chromosomes. Mitosis, in contrast, produces two nuclei each containing the diploid number of chromosomes. Furthermore, each daughter nucleus produced by mitosis contains an identical set of chromosomes and therefore genes to that possessed by the original undivided cell. Meiosis, on the

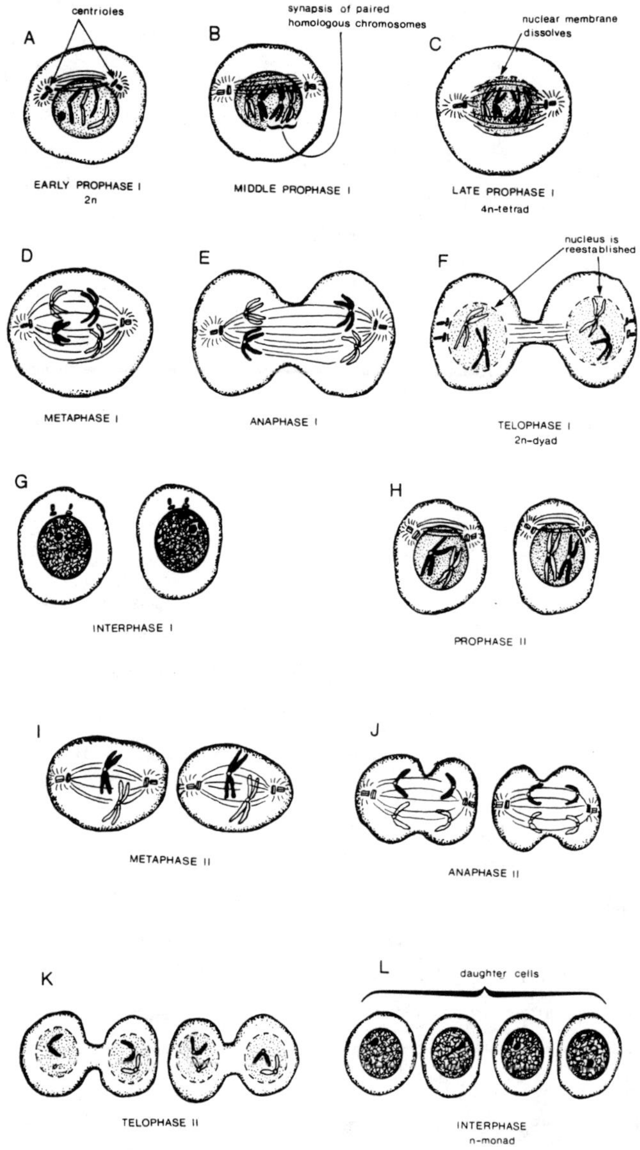

other hand, produces four daughter nuclei that are genetically *different* from each other and from the parent nucleus.

As meiosis begins, the chromosomes replicate themselves in the same way as occurs in mitosis. Each chromosome thus consists of two idential chromatids held together by a kinetochore. As meiotic *prophase* comes to a close, the nuclear membrane breaks down (as it does in mitosis). Unlike the situation in mitosis, however, the chromosomes do not line up in a single line along the equatorial plane. Instead, they come together in *homologous pairs* (each pair consisting of the corresponding chromosome from each parent). Thus, maternal chromosome 21 comes to lie alongside paternal chromosome 21, the two sex chromosomes similarly pair up and so on. Because each chromosome in the homologous pair sets has already duplicated itself into two daughter chromatids, each homologous pair consists of four chromatids. These four-stranded synaptic pairs are referred to as *tetrads*. The tetrads then separate during *anaphase*, one replicated chromosome from each homologous pair going to opposite sides of the cell, each being pulled away by spindle fibers attached to its kinetochore. Because the kinetochores have not divided, the two chromatids of each replicated chromosome remain together, unlike the situation in mitosis. The cell then divides and enters a "resting" stage called *interphase*.

Each daughter cell now contains one replicated chromosome from each homologous pair. This means that each daughter cell contains a complement of 22 autosomes and one sex chromosome, one from each parent. As the homologous pairs come together at the equatorial plane, the chromosomes from each parent do not necessarily all line up on the same side. Thus each daughter cell is likely to receive some chromosomes from each parent. Chromosome 21 in a given daughter cell, for example, may be maternal, chromosome 13 paternal, and so forth. Furthermore, while the homologous pairs are lined up together along the equatorial plane, *crossing over* or *translocation* frequently takes place in which portions of the chromatid from one member of a homologous pair will fuse with its counterpart from the other member of the pair. Thus, the homologous pair may actually exchange portions of their chromosomes, so that the chromatid tip which originally belonged to one member of the pair becomes broken off and becomes attached to the other pair member. And conversely, the tip from the other member of the pair detaches and becomes part of the first pair member.

Because the allele pairs of the homologous pair all lie in exactly the same corresponding place on each chromosome of the pair, such crossing over still provides that each member of the homologous pair will contain all the genes normally found on that chromosome. It is clear, therefore, that because of the independent assortment of the members of each homologous pair to the daughter cells, and because of the tendency for crossing over to occur during *metaphase I* in meiosis, there is essentially no limit to the possible combinations of genes each daughter cell product of the first meiotic division may receive.

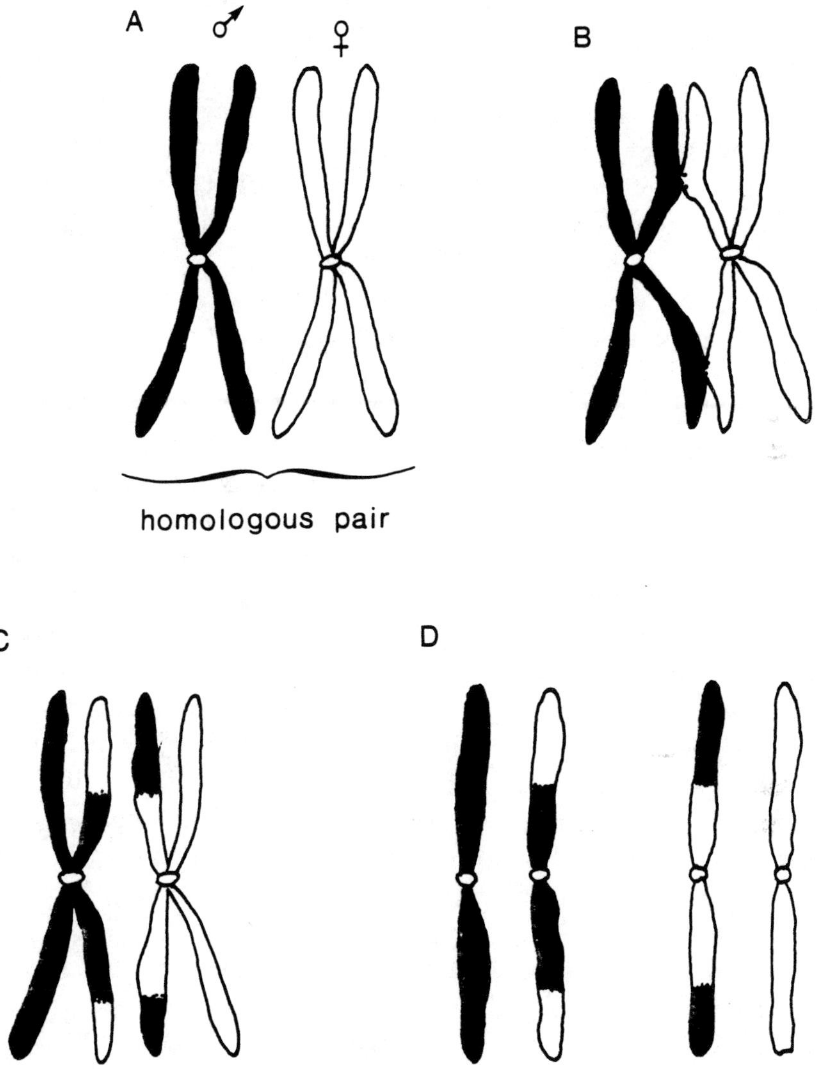

At the end of the first meiotic division each daughter nucleus contains one-half the number of chromosomes originally present during the *4n-tetrad* stage of prophase I. Each daughter nucleus now has a *2n-dyad* number of chromosomes.

During the second meiotic division, which closely resembles mitosis, the nuclear membrane again disappears and each of the 2n-dyad (replicated chromosomes line up along the equatorial plane—this time in single file as in mitosis. The kinetochores divide and each chromatid, now a single chromosome, is pulled by the spindle fiber system toward opposite poles of the cell. The cytoplasm constricts in the middle and *cytokinesis* and cell division follow. Each daughter cell resulting from meiosis I has now itself given rise to two daughter cells, each with the haploid or *n-monad* number of chromosomes.

In fact, during human gametogenesis, each diploid *spermatogonium* undergoes chromosome replication to form a 4n-tetrad primary *spermatocyte.* Each primary spermatocyte then undergoes the first meiotic division to become two 2n-dyad *secondary spermatocytes.* These, in turn, undergo the second meiotic division to form four n-monad or haploid spermatids which then grow tails and undergo other cytoplasmic transformations to become four haploid and motile *spermatozoa.* In the maturation of the human egg, the diploid *oogonium* undergoes chromosome replication to become a *primary oocyte.* The primary oocyte then undergoes the first reduction division to form a 2n-dyad *secondary oocyte* and an n-dyad *polar body* (the polar body is the nuclear equivalent of the secondary oocyte without the cytoplasm). The female ova are present in the female very early during fetal development, and the first reduction division typically occurs in humans during the third gestational month. The secondary oocyte and the first polar body do not undergo the second meiotic division until and unless fertilization occurs many years later at sexual maturity. When that occurs, the secondary oocyte produces an n-monad or haploid *ovum* or egg ready for fertilization, plus a haploid polar body. Likewise the first polar body produces two additional haploid polar bodies. Of the four haploid nuclear products of meiosis in the developing human ovum, only one functional haploid egg is produced; the three polar bodies disintegrate. When a haploid spermatozoon and a haploid ovum come together, the nuclei fuse and a diploid zygote is produced.

Meiosis thus results in daughter cells quite different from the parent cell both in chromosome number and chromosome composition because of independent segregation and crossing over. Whereas mitosis guarantees genetic sameness, meiosis guarantees genetic heterogeneity and diversity. Each child derives half of his or her chromosomes from each parent. But because the parental gametes undergo the process of meiosis, the egg and sperm produced can have almost any combination of genes from the child's parents, with the sole proviso being that every gene is represented by one allele in each gamete.

In 1865, the Austrian monk, Gregor Mendel, founded the science of genetics when he published the results of his breeding experiments with peas. He also provided a model for the variation existing in organisms to account for the evolution of new life forms out of previously existing ones as described in Charles Darwin's publication of his bombshell in 1859—*The Origin of Species.*

Mendel found that different varieties of peas always bred true: for example plants with yellow flowers always produced yellow-flowered progeny, tall plants gave rise to tall progeny, and so forth. However, when he crossbred different varieties of peas with each other, some of the traits disappeared completely in the first filial or *F_1 generation.* For example, breeding true-breeding yellow-seeded plants with true-breeding green-seeded plants produced only yellow-seeded progeny. And crossing true-breeding tall plants with true-breeding short plants produced an F_1 generation consisting only of tall plants. Mendel referred to those alternate traits that are universally expressed in the F_1 generation arising from a cross between two different varieties as being *dominant;* those traits that are totally suppressed in the F_1 generation he called *recessive.* Thus, tall plants with yellow seeds will always emerge and dwarf plants with green seeds will never appear in the F_1 generation arising out of a cross between the two types.

If F_1 plants are crossed with each other, the recessive traits that had disappeared reappeared in the F_2 generation in the ratio of three dominant progeny to every one recessive. Mendel realized that the factors for each trait must *segregate independently* during the production of gametes, and that these factors must be discrete. These factors must also occur in pairs in each organism and one of each pair must be inherited from each parent. These factors are then again segregated during germ cell production by the F_1 generation plants, one factor of the pair going to each of the two kinds of gametes produced. This is known as Mendel's first law, the *law* or *principle of segregation.* The factors for alternating traits became known as *genes,* for example, genes for plant height or seed color. The individual varieties of each gene are *alleles,* for example, the gene for plant height has two alleles (in this example), one of which produces tall plants and the other short ones. When both alleles for a given trait are identical, the organism is said to be *homozygous* for that trait; when the alleles are different, the organism is *heterozygous* for that trait. (Heterozygous individuals are sometimes referred to as hybrids, but this term can be misleading since it also, and probably more appropriately, refers to crosses between different races, subspecies, and even species in some cases.)[74] The actual genetic makeup of an organism is its *genotype* whereas its outward appearance is its *phenotype.*

Mendel's experiments produced a clear consistency in the inheritance

[74]A biological species is generally defined as a taxonomic population that maintains its genetic integrity, i.e., does not outbreed with other taxonomic populations. While this is a reasonably good working definition, many full species do interbreed regularly (domestic dogs with coyotes and wolves; it is especially common among reptiles).

ratio of three dominant phenotypes to every recessive phenotype when homozygous plants with contrasting traits were crossbred. Thus, he got 787 tall plants to 277 short plants, 6,022 yellow-seeded plants to 2,001 green-seeded ones, 705 red-flowered plants to 224 white-flowered ones, and so forth. Simple arithmetic shows that these are ratios of 2.84, 3.01 and 3.15, respectively.

A useful way to examine the manner in which alternate traits are passed from one generation to another is by use of the *Punnett square.* In the case of tall and dwarf pea plants, the plants homozygous for the dominant (tall) allele are designated as TT, that is they have one tall allele from each parent. The homozygous recessive plants are designated as tt. Both of these homozygotes can only produce one kind of gamete. Thus in a cross between the two the dominant homozygotes will produce only *T* gametes and the recessive homozygotes only *t* gametes. All of the F_1 progeny will therefore have a *Tt* genotype and express the dominant (tall) phenotype. If the F_1 generation plants are self-fertilized, each plant will produce both *T-* and *t*-bearing gametes, and the possible combinations that will be produced in the F_2 generation are:

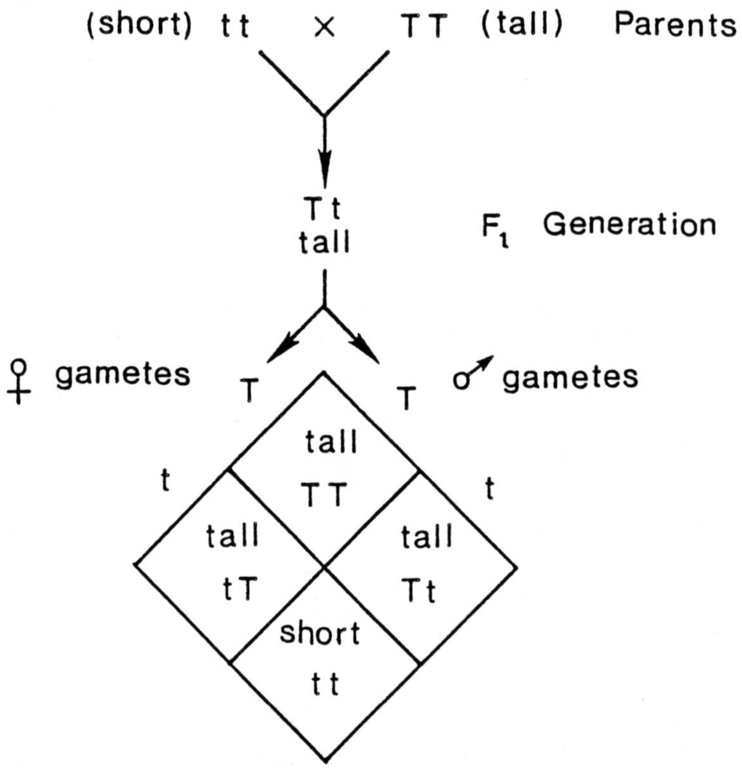

The F_2 genotypes thus include one dominant *TT* homozygote, two *Tt* heterozygotes and one recessive *tt* homozygote for every four F_2 plants produced. This gives a ratio of three tall phenotypes to every one short phenotype when alternate traits are considered separately. When crossing dominant and recessive homozygous parents, the recessive phenotype will always be completely suppressed in the F_1 generation, only to reappear in the F_2 generation. At most loci, however, there are more than just two alleles, and most if not all loci are *polyallelic*. This, of course, greatly increases the possible genetic variability in the offspring. A locus with just two alleles can produce three different genotypes, one with three alleles can produce six genotypes, and one with six different alleles can produce 21 different genotypes.

When two loci are considered together, for example plant size and flower color, the recessive phenotypes will again be suppressed in the F_1 generation and reappear in the F_2. This time, however, not only will both dominant and recessive phenotypes appear, but totally new combinations of traits representing a mixture of the features of the parents. For example, crossing two homozygous parents with the genotypes *TTRR* (tall and red-flowered) and *ttrr* (short and white) will yield:

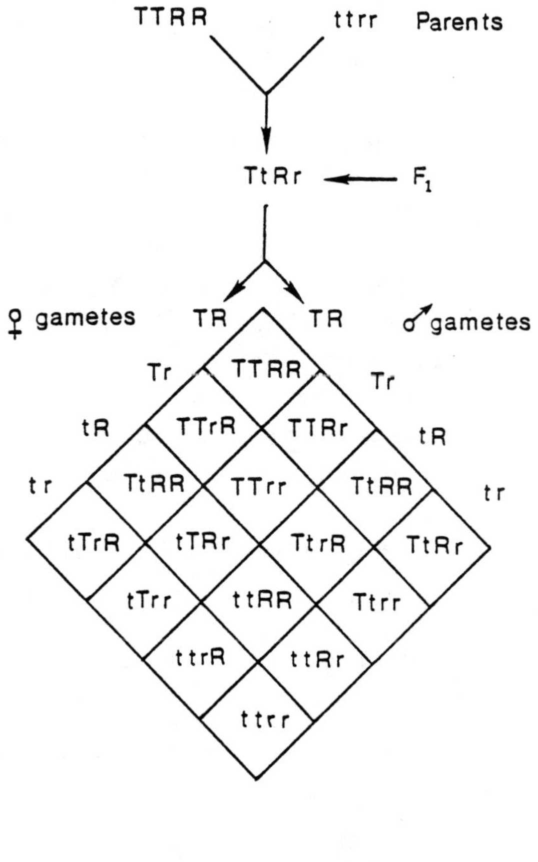

From the Punnett square it can be seen that the F_2 generation will produce nine tall, red plants, three tall, white ones, three short, red ones, and one short, white one. A cross involving two pairs of alleles will produce this 9:3:3:1 ratio whether one of the parents is homozygous for both recessive traits and the other homozygous dominant, or each parent is homozygous for one dominant and one recessive trait *(TTrr × ttRR)*.

Frequently, the combination of two different alleles results in a blending of the two traits to produce an intermediate phenotype—a phenomenon known as *incomplete dominance.* For example, a cross between certain red and white cattle produces one red homozygous animal, two intermediate, roan-colored, heterozygous animals and one homozygous white animal in a 1:2:1 ratio (Baker and Allen 1979). Similarly, crossing a red snapdragon with a white one produces one red homozygote (*RR*), one white homozygote (*rr*) and two intermediate, pink heterozygotes (*Rr*) (Curtis 1972). Some genes also exhibit *intermediate inheritance*—that is, single dominant automsome transmission in which all the homozygotes but only some of the heterozygotes express the dominant phenotype. *Codominance* may also occur as given by the example on page 35 in which crosses between the alleles I^A and I^B result in the human blood type AB where both alleles are equally manifested by the phenotype.

Genes which lie on the same chromosome do not show the rule of independent transmission described above, and will always be transmitted together in a given germ cell. This is known as *linkage.* Because of crossing over at meiosis, however, genes formerly on one chromosome may end up on the other member of the homologous pair and thus find themselves in different gametes. This process is called *recombination.* The farther apart two genes are from one another on a given chromosome, the greater is the likelihood that they may be separated during crossing over events. The closer together, the more likely both are to be recombined together with the same fragment of chromosome. Because of this, geneticists are able to mathematically determine the locations of genes along a chromosome by the degree of linkage and independent recombination they exhibit.

In the case where a gene is represented by two different alleles in the general population, we can let p = the frequency of allele A and q = the frequency of allele a. The frequencies of these two alleles taken together must equal the frequency of the gene as a whole, that is 100 percent. Therefore, if 90 percent of the alleles in the population are A, and there are only two alleles, then allele a must comprise ten percent and the two together = 100 percent. This can be expressed mathematically as $.9 + .1 = 1.0$; therefore $p + q = 1$. When we square both sides of the equation we obtain $(p + q)^2 = (1)^2 = 1$, and by expanding the binomial we get $p^2 + 2pq + q^2 = 1$. In the example just given $p = .9$ and $q = .1$, and when we substitute these numbers into the equation we get $(.81 + .18 + .01) = 1$. This relationship is known as the *Hardy-Weinberg relationship* and it describes the frequency of genotypes that would be produced by random mating within the population of alleles under consideration. In the absence of selective pressures (i.e., the alleles are both selectively neutral) and other disturbing influences (e.g. population migrations), the gene frequencies will remain the same and the genotypes will occur in the relative frequencies p^2, $2pq$, and q^2 through all subsequent generations. This relationship can also be represented in a Punnett square:

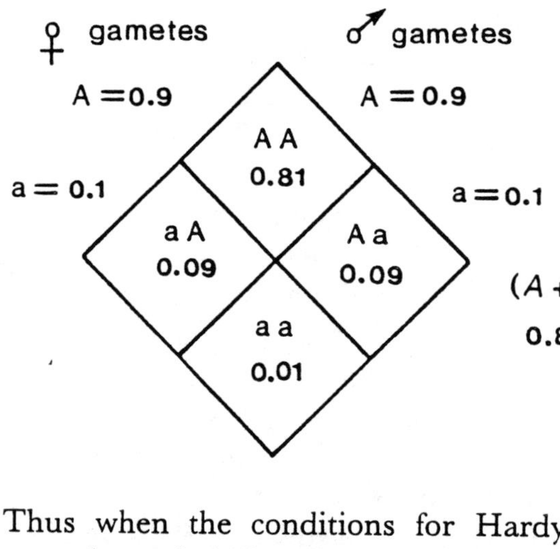

$$(A + a)^2 = A^2 + 2Aa + a^2$$
$$0.81 + 2(0.09) + 0.1 = 1$$

Thus when the conditions for Hardy-Weinberg equilibrium are present, the probability of getting genotype *AA* in the foregoing example is .81 (81%), of getting genotype *Aa* is .18 (18%) and of obtaining genotype *aa* is .01 (1%). When three alleles at one locus are being considered, the Hardy-Weinberg formula becomes $(p + q + r)^2 = 1$. In order for Hardy-Weinberg equilibrium to apply, several conditions must be met:

(1) Mating in the population must be random (i.e., no sexual or other selection).

(2) All matings must produce approximately equal numbers of offspring.

(3) The mutation rates between alleles must have attained equilibrium—that is the rate of mutation from allele $A \rightarrow$ allele a must

equal the number of back mutations from allele $a \rightarrow$ allele A.[75]

(4) The populations must be very large so that random variations do not significantly affect the gene frequencies.

(5) There is no significant migration into or out of the population.

(6) There is no significant selective pressure for or against the trait, i.e., the trait is evolutionarily neutral.

All of these conditions rarely exist in any given case, but the theoretical Hardy-Weinberg equilibrium model is a powerful formulation of the dynamics of population genetics and it specifies the kinds of factors that oppose that equilibrium. One such factor is *assortative mating,* a deviation from random mating in which like individuals preferentially mate with each other (*positive assortative mating*) or unlike individuals preferentially mate (*negative assortative mating*). This is somewhat similar to *sexual selection,* in which certain genotypes in the male and/or female are selected for. Theoretically, assortative mating differs from sexual selection in that the former does not result in changes in gene frequencies whereas such changes occur in the latter. In practice, assortative mating that is completely divorced from changes in gene frequencies is probably rarely achieved.

There are several different consequences due to assortative mating. Positive assortative mating for a recessive phenotype, such as deafness, tends to increase the frequency of that phenotype. The tendency of deaf people to marry other deaf people produces a greater number of recessive, homozygous deaf offspring, although it does not affect the actual gene frequency for deafness in the population. In modern, civilized society there is little selection against the survival of handicapped individuals and their numbers would tend to increase.

Assortative mating for polygenic traits exaggerates the additive portion of the variance or difference between the homozygotes for various genes. Additivity refers to the assumption that the effects of all the genes involved in a polygenic trait are simply summed. This assumption may or may not be correct in any given case. Positive assortative mating tends to increase the number of homozygous genotypes for a polygenic trait over that produced by random mating within the general population. As a result there is an increase in the frequency of individuals who bear the extreme expressions of such traits. Assortative mating may have significant effects upon the phenotypic expression of psychiatric disor-

[75] Although mutations, particularly point mutations, are largely random events, certain specific mutations of one allele into another and back again occur with a regular frequency.

ders, since psychiatrically ill persons tend to marry others with psychiatric disorders. This is particularly true of alcoholics and co-alcoholics and those with serious personality disorders, especially histrionic and sociopathic personality disorders.

APPENDIX II

THE CENTRAL nervous system in vertebrate animals begins as two parallel ridges of neural ectoderm (see Figure 20C-D) which emerge from the uppermost or dorsal surface of the developing embryo.[76] These two ridges then fuse along their lengths, forming an elongated, hollow neural tube (Figure 20E-F). As development proceeds, a series of expanded chambers connected by constrictions form along the length of the neural tube (Figure 31), dividing the presumptive central nervous system into three major sections: the *prosencephalon, mesencephalon* and *rhombencephalon,* corresponding to the *forebrain, midbrain* and *hindbrain,* respectively. The *prosencephalon* then subdivides into the *telencephalon* and the *diencephalon,* and the *rhombencephalon* gives rise to the *metencephalon* and the *myelencephalon* (Figure 31A).

The telencephalon develops into two large, side-by-side chambers known as the *first* and *second ventricles.* The walls of these chambers are destined to become the two cerebral hemispheres of the adult brain — the portion of the CNS associated with consciousness, learning and reasoning. The floor of the first two ventricles gives rise to the *basal ganglia* and elements of the *limbic system,* which mediate the experience and regulation of emotion. Projecting forward from the cerebral hemispheres are two *olfactory bulbs* which continue to subserve a prominent sensory role in lower vertebrates, including many mammals, but which in man have lost much of their former function. The olfactory bulbs and their attached *olfactory tubercles* (Figures 31-33) remain an integral part of the limbic system in man, and are partly responsible for the powerful feelings of *déjà vu* which we all experience from time to time associated with odors which are either real or hallucinatory, and which evoke powerful emotional states associated with some early experience we can never really quite place.

[76]The material in this appendix has been largely reproduced from an earlier volume in this series (Light 1986a, pages 46-52); the reader is referred there for a detailed discussion of central nervous system structure and function.

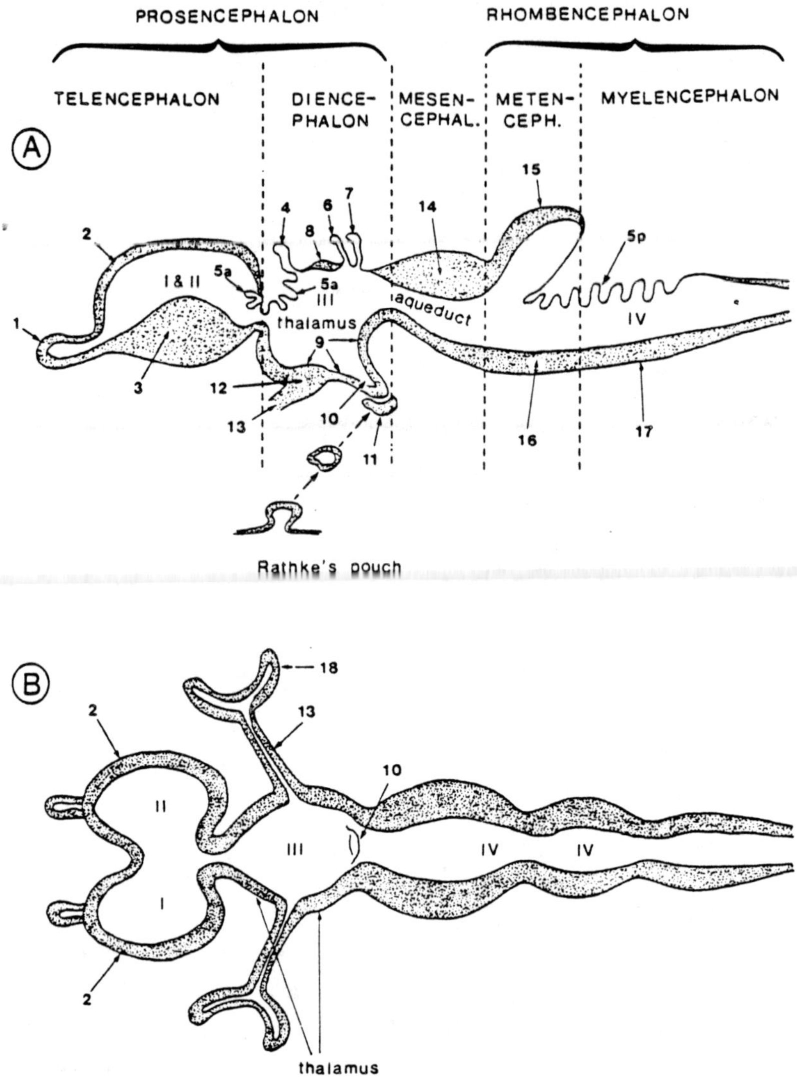

Figure 31. Embryonic Divisions of the Brain. A. A median longitudinal section through the embryonic brain. The three major divisions of the brain, the prosencephalon, mesencephalon and rhombencephalon, correspond to the forebrain, midbrain and hindbrain, respectively. 1 = olfactory tubercle; 2 = cerebral hemispheres; 3 = floor of telencephalon which gives rise to the paired basal ganglia of the adult brain; 4 = paraphysis, a structure of obscure function; 5a = anterior choroid plexus; 5b = posterior choroid plexus; 6 = parapineal (parietal organ); 7 = epiphysis (pineal body); 8 = epithalamus; 9 = hypothalamus; 10 = infundibulum; 11 = adenohypophysis (anterior lobe of pituitary) derived from Rathke's pouch; 12 = optic chiasma; 13 = optic tract; 14 = tectum; 15 = cerebellum; 16 = pons; 17 = medulla oblongata. **B.** Overhead or dorsal view of plane section through the embryonic brain. The numbers are the same as in A. 18 = developing retinal cup of the eye (see also Figure 32), a structure deriving directly as a lateral outgrowth of the diencephalon. Roman numerals indicate the various ventricles of the brain in both A and B. From Light 1986a, Figure 16.

The diencephalon encloses the *third ventricle* of the brain. The side walls of the diencephalon comprise the paired *thalami,* which play a major role in relaying incoming and outgoing information to appropriate centers for assessment and action; they also function in motor control. The floor of the diencephalon becomes the *hypothalamus* which mediates the expression of emotion and which contains the neural centers controlling a variety of physiological drives, such as sexuality, hunger, thirst, and satiety. A prominent ventral (downward) outpocket of the hypothalamus is termed the *infundibulum* (Figure 31); it will form the posterior lobe of the pituitary gland—the *neurohypophysis.* The anterior lobe of the pituitary—the *adenohypophysis*—derives from *Rathke's pouch,* a diverticulum which pinches off from the roof of the pharynx and migrates to and fuses with the infundibulum (Figure 31A). The *optic chiasma* also arises within the hypothalamus just anterior to the pituitary complex; this structure marks the point at which the optic fibers from the eyeballs enter the main part of the brain, half of the fibers from each tract crossing over into the opposite side of the brain. The optic nerves and retinae of the eyes are themselves thus formed from direct outpockets of the diencephalon (Figures 31 and 32) and are thus true extensions of the brain. Just posterior to the infundibulum, the hypothalamus gives rise to two ventral protuberances known as the *mammillary bodies* (Figure 34). These nuclei are involved in memory functions and in the expression of rage.

The roof of the diencephalon—the *epithelamus*—gives rise to two glandular bodies known as the *parietal* and *pineal bodies,* which served as a functional pair of median eyes in ancient vertebrates (see Light 1986a, footnote 24). The pineal body persists in higher vertebrates today as a light-sensitive endocrine organ which is directly influenced by seasonal changes in the daylight to darkness ratio, and it regulates the release of hormones from the hypothalamus which affect the anterior lobe of the pituitary. In humans, *melatonin* is synthesized from serotonin (an important neurotransmitter in the brain) in the pineal gland, which plays an important role in the sleep-wake cycle.

The brain is largely surrounded by thick walls of neural tissue except for two regions: (1) the junction between the roof of the telencephalon and that of the anterior part of the epithalamus, and (2) the roof of the fourth ventricle—the expanded part of the neural cavity lying behind the third ventricle (Figures 31 and 33). Each of these two regions has a thin, folded, and curtainlike tissue richly supplied with blood vessels known as the *anterior* and *posterior choroid plexi* (singular, *plexus)* respectively. The choroid plexi are regions where an exchange of materials

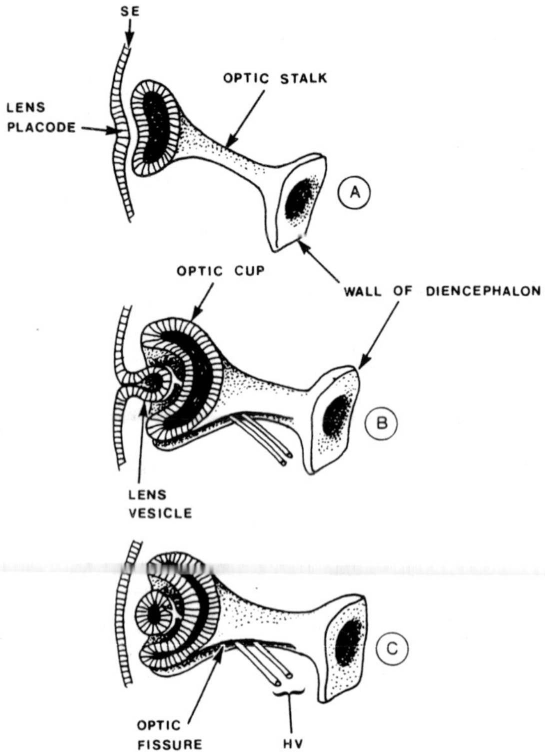

Figure 32. Formation of the Eye. A, B, and C. Schematic sections of the developing eye showing the differentiation of the optic cup and lens vesicle. The lens vesicle is induced from the head ectoderm by the optic cup. HV = hyaloid vessels (artery and vein). Adapted and modified from Moore 1973, Figure 19-1.

occurs between the blood and the *cerebrospinal fluid* within the brain's ventricles. The blood-brain barrier (see Light 1986a) is compromised in this region and a variety of foreign substances, including many drugs, has ready access to the brain itself.

The third and fourth ventricles are connected by the *aqueduct of Sylvius,* and the thick roof overlying the aqueduct is the *tectum,* which bears four small mounds known as the *corpora quadrigemina* that integrate visual and auditory signals coming into the brain.

The *cerebellum* develops from the roof of the metencephalon. This is a complex structure containing a rich "reverberating" neuronal circuitry (see Light 1986a) which functions in the coordination and regulation of motor activity and in the maintenance of balance and posture. It is readily affected by a variety of drugs, especially alcohol, which produces the ataxia or loss of coordination seen in intoxicated states. The floor of the metencephalon develops into the *pons* (Figures 33 and 34) which is a major pathway for ascending and descending fibers between the brain and the spinal cord. The *reticular formation*—the seat of consciousness arousal—is located in the pons as well as in the lower-lying *medulla oblongata*; consciousness is maintained via a complex system of ascending nerve tracts to the higher cortex known as the *reticular activating system.* The medulla oblongata is essentially an expanded version of the spinal cord, but it houses many important nerve centers involved in the control of blood pressure, heart rate, breathing, and vomiting. When drug-induced central depression begins to affect these medullary centers, the intoxicated person stands a good chance of losing his or her life.

In humans, the primitive, embryonic brain structures just described undergo major changes in the configurations of and the relationships between these elements. Because humans walk upright, the orientation of the brain structures is from top to bottom, rather than fore to aft as in most quadrupeds. The human brainstem has become a vertical mushroomlike structure crowned by the hypothalamus and paired thalmi of the diencephalon (Figure 33). The basal ganglia derived from the floor of the telencephalon now surround the diencephalon. The paired lateral ventricles (I and II) project approximately laterally from the level of the diencephalon, and are themselves enclosed within the two massive cerebral hemispheres.

In primitive vertebrates the telencephalon is closely associated with the development of the olfactory lobes, and the cerebral hemispheres are mainly concerned with integrating and processing olfactory signals. The cerebral cortex at this stage of evolutionary development is known as the *paleocortex* (or paleopallium)—the "ancient" cortex. In higher vertebrates such as reptiles the paleocortex is restricted to the lower sidewalls and floor of the telencephalon. This paleocortical region gives rise to the basal ganglia of the limbic system in reptiles and mammals. Above the paleocortex and towards the center of the cerebral hemispheres lies the *archicortex* (or archipallium)—the "old" cortex. This region gives rise to the *hippocampus* in mammals (Figure 34) by a recurved folding of the inner, medial part of the temporal lobes. The hippocampus is intimately involved in memory and learning, and toxic insult to this region, as occurs with alcoholic Wernicke-Korsakoff psychosis, results in profound memory impairment. The paleocortex and archicortex and their derivatives are often referred to as the "reptilian brain." These regions are closely associated with emotion in the higher mammals.

The cerebral hemispheres, most of which comprise the *neocortex* (neopallium) or "new" brain, cover the entire brain as paired, massive,

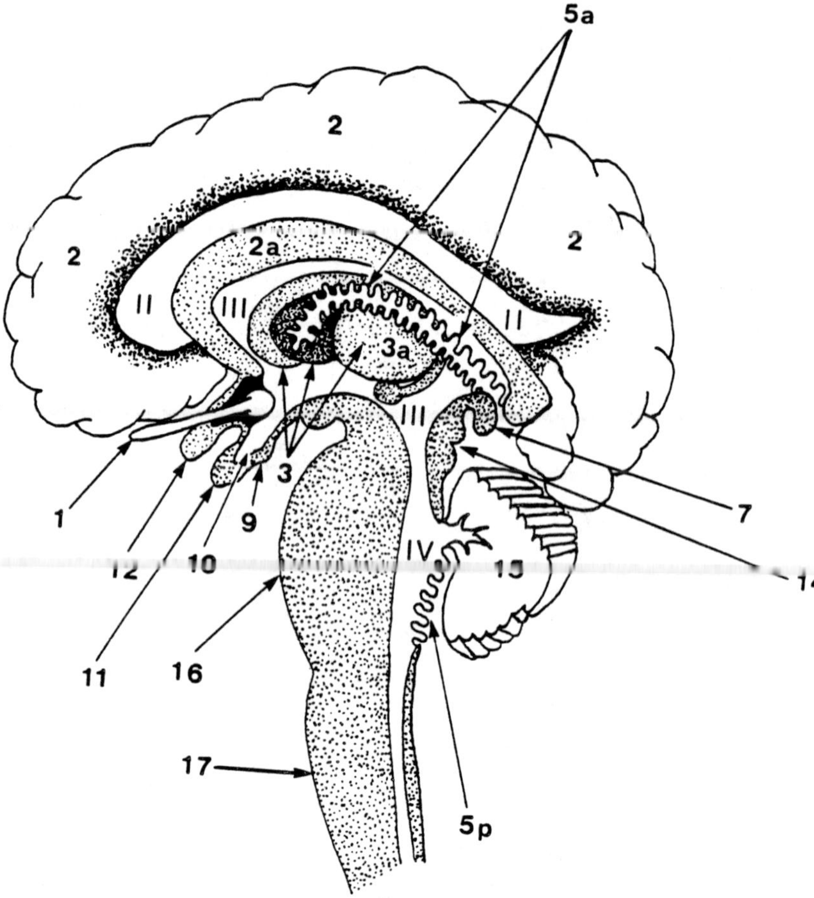

Figure 33. Human Brain: Median Longitudinal Section I. In this figure of the adult human brain, the basic structures in Figure 31 are shown here as collapsed back upon the brainstem with the cerebral hemispheres flanking the diencephalon on each side. The thalamus is now restricted to two reduced ganglia flanking the now considerably compressed third ventricle. The other basal ganglia are derived from the floor of the telencephalon. The olfactory bulbs and tubercles are considerably reduced from the embryonic condition and they are allied and interconnected with the amygdala of the limbic system. The numbers are the same as in Figure 31, except that 3 = the basal ganglia, including the thalamus, and 3a = the thalamus itself. The tectum (14) is shown here as the four mounded nuclei of the corpora quadrigemina, which are involved in the processing of visual and auditory stimuli. From Light 1986a, Figure 17.

and highly convoluted globes which have grown forward, laterally, and rearward to cap the limbic structures, diencephalon, and the midbrain region like the top of a huge mushroom (Figures 33 and 34). The advanced brains of mammals and particularly of humans are thus arranged in a series of concentric shells, with the evolutionarily and embryologically most advanced and recently differentiated shells encapsulating the earlier, more primitive regions.[77] The limbic system formed from the reptilian brain, together with the hypothalamus derived from

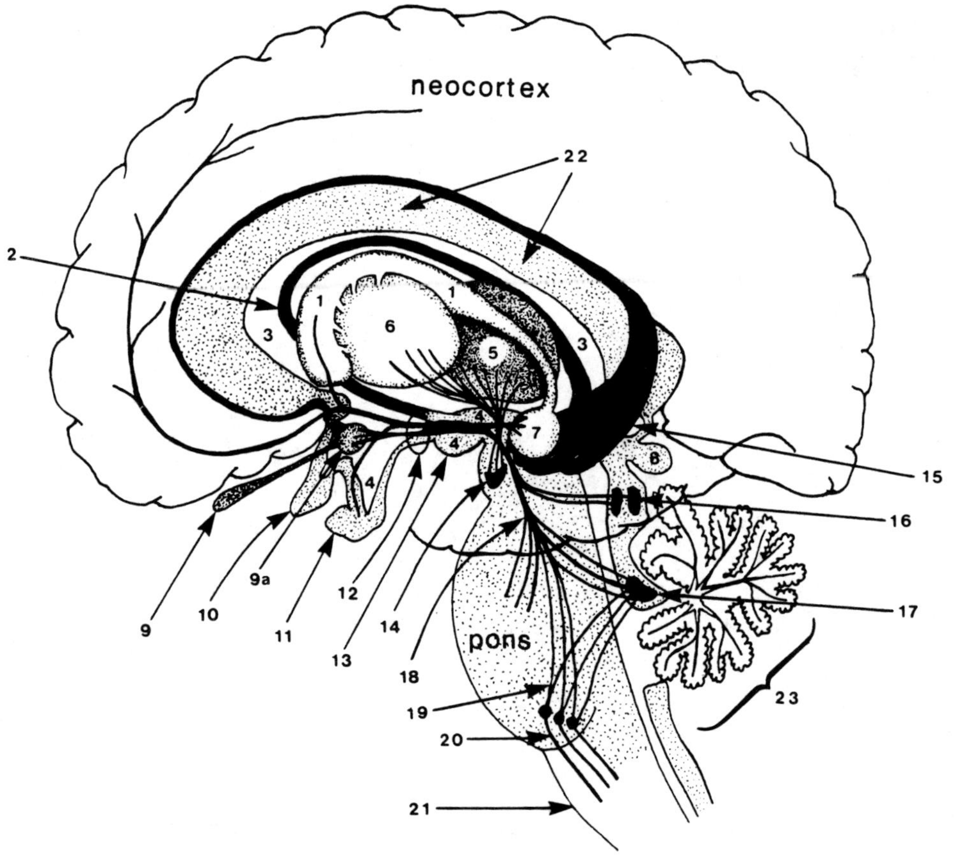

Figure 34. Human Brain: Median Longitudinal Section II. 1 = caudate nucleus; 2 = fornix; 3 = third ventricle; 4 = hypothalamus; 5 = thalamus; 6 = corpus striatum (putamen and globus pallidus); 7 = amygdala; 8 = pineal gland; 9 = olfactory bulb; 10 = optic chiasma; 11 = anterior lobe of pituitary (adenohypophysis); 12 = medial forebrain bundle; 13 = mammillary body; 14 = substantia nigra; 15 = hippocampus; 16 = raphe nuclei; 17 = locus coeruleus; 18 = ascending tracts from locus coeruleus; 19 = interconnecting nerves between locus coeruleus and ascending and descending tracts; 20 = descending tracts from locus coeruleus; 21 = medulla oblongata; 22 = corpus callosum; 23 = cerebellum. From Light 1986a, Figure 19.

[77]In the nineteenth century, the noted German naturalist-philospher made his famous statement that "ontogeny recapitulates phylogeny." By this he meant that during its embryonic development, an organism undergoes the same sequence of morphological changes as its ancestors manifested during their evolution from lower to higher life forms. Although this dictum is by no means as universally applicable as was once believed, it nevertheless contains more than an element of truth. It is evidenced, for example, in the development of transient gill arches and tails in the embryogenesis of mammals, including human beings, which reflect the evolutionary changes which occurred in the evolution of the vertebrates from ancestral fishes through amphibians and reptiles to modern mammals.

the floor of the diencephalon mediate the experience and expression of emotional states, particularly rage and aggression. These primitive functions are modified, channeled, and inhibited by the surrounding outer shell of the neocortex. The reader is referred to a previous volume in this series (Light 1986a) for a more detailed discussion of the brain and its functioning in adult human beings.

BIBLIOGRAPHY

Amark, C.: A study in alcoholism. *Acta Psychiat. Scand., Suppl.* 70: 1-283, 1951.

American Psychiatric Association: *Diagnostic and Statistical Manual of Mental Disorders,* Third Edition. Washington, D.C., 1980.

Arey, L.B.: *Developmental Anatomy: A Textbook and Laboratory Manual of Embryology.* Philadelphia: W.B. Saunders, 1965.

Beck, E.C., Dustman, R.E., Blusewicz, T., Schenkenberg, T., and Cannon, W.G.: Cerebral evoked potentials and correlated neuropsychological changes in the human brain during aging: a comparison of alcoholism and aging. In Ordy, J.M., and Brizzee, K.R. (Eds.): *Aging: Sensory Systems and Information Processing.* New York: Raven Press, 1978, pp. 203-226.

Begleiter, H., Porjesz, B., Bihari, B., and Kissin, B.: Event-related brain potentials in boys at risk for alcoholism. *Science 225:* 1493-1496, 1984.

Begleiter, H., Porjesz, B., and Chou, C.L.: Auditory brainstem potentials in chronic alcoholics. *Science 211:* 1064-1066.

Beskid, M., Majdecki, T., and Skladzinski, J.: The effect of ethanol applied during gestation on the mitochondria of the hepatic cells of pups. *Folia Histochem. Cytochem. 13:* 175-180, 1975.

Bishop, J.M.: Oncogenes. *Sci. Amer. 246:* 80-92.

Blum, K., Eubanks, J.D., Wallace, J.E., Schwertner, H., and Morgan, W.W.: Possible role of tetrahydroisoquinoline alkaloids in postalcohol intoxication states. *Annals N. Y. Acad. Sci. 273:* 234-246, 1976.

Bowman, W.C., and Rand, M.J.: *Textbook of Pharmacology, Second Edition.* Oxford: Blackwell Scientific Publications, 1980.

Buchsbaum, M.S.: Averaged evoked response and stimulus intensity in identical and fraternal twins. *Physiol. Psychol. 2:* 365-370, 1974.

Buchsbaum, M.S.: Appendix E. Neurophysiological studies of reduction and augmentation. In Petrie, A.: *Individuality in Pain and Suffering.* Chicago: University of Chicago Press, 1978, pp. 141-155.

Burtle, V.: *Women Who Drink: Alcoholic Experience and Psychotherapy.* Springfield: Charles C Thomas, 1979.

Cadoret, R.J., Cain, C.A., and Grove, W.M.: Development of alcoholism in adoptees raised apart from alcoholic biologic relatives. *Arch. Gen. Psych. 37:*561-563, 1980.

Cahalan, D., Cisin, I.H., and Crossley, H.M.: *American Drinking Practices: A National Study of Drinking Behavior and Attitudes.* New Haven: College and University Press, 1969.

Camberwell Council on Alcoholism: *Women and Alcohol.* London and New York: Tavistock Publications, 1980.

Chernoff, G.F.: Introduction: A teratologist's view of the fetal alcohol syndrome. In Galanter, M. (Ed.): *Currents in Alcoholism. Vol. VII. Recent Advances in Research and Treatment.* New York: Grune and Stratton, 1980, pp. 7-13.

Cloninger, R.C., Bohman, M., and Sigvardsson, S.: Inheritance of alcohol abuse: cross-fostering analysis of adopted men. *Arch. Gen. Psychiat. 38:* 861-868, 1981.

Cloninger, R.C., and Reich, T.: Genetic heterogeneity in alcoholism and sociopathy. In Kety, S.S., Rowland, L.P., Sidman, R.L., and Matthysse, S.W.: *Genetics of Neurological and Psychiatric Disorders.* New York: Raven Press, 1983, pp. 145-166.

Cloninger, R.C., Reich, T., and Wetzel, R.: Alcoholism and affective disorders: familial associations and genetic models. In Goodwin, D.W., and Erickson, C.K. (Eds.): *Alcoholism and Affective Disorders: Clinical, Genetic and Biochemical Studies.* New York: SP Medical and Scientific Books, 1979, pp. 57-86.

Cohen, G.: Interaction of catecholeamines with acetaldehyde to form tetrahydroisoquinoline neurotransmitters. In Sharp, C.W., and Abood, L.G. (Eds.): *Progress in Clinical and Biological Research.* New York: Alan R. Liss, 1979, pp. 73-90.

Corrigan, F. M.: *Alcoholic Women in Treatment.* New York and Oxford: Oxford University Press, 1980.

Cruz-Coke, R., and Varela, A.: Inheritance of alcoholism: its association with colour-blindness. *Lancet ii:* 1282-1284, 1966.

Davis, V.E., and Walsh, M.J.: Alcohol, amines and alkaloids: a possible biochemical basis for alcohol addiction. *Science 167:* 1005-1007, 1970.

Dustman, R.E., Snyder, W.W., Calner, D.A., and Beck, E.C.: The evoked response as a measure of cerebral dysfunction. In Begleiter, H. (Ed.): *Evoked Brain Potentials and Behavior.* Vol. 2. New York: Plenum Press, 1979, pp. 321-364.

Ehrmann, L., and Parsons, P.A.: *The Genetics of Behavior.* Sunderland, MA: Sinauer Associates, Inc., 1976.

Fernhof, P.M.: *Family Practice News 13*(23): 1, 1983.

Fine, E.W., Richman, S.A., and Teichman, M.: Depression in female alcoholics. In Galanter, M. (Ed.): *Currents in Alcoholism. Vol. VII. Recent Advances in Research and Treatment.* New York: Grune and Stratton, 1980, pp. 447-453.

Ghodse, A.H., and Tregenza, G.S.: The physical effects and metabolism of alcohol. In Camberwell Council on Alcoholism: *Women and Alcohol.* London and New York: Tavistock Publications, 1980, pp. 41-52.

Gomberg, E.S.: The female alcoholic. In Tartar, R.E., and Sugarman, A.A.: *Alcoholism: Interdisciplinary Approaches to an Enduring Problem.* Reading, MA: Addison-Wesley, 1976, pp. 603-636.

Gomberg, E.S.: Drinking patterns of women alcoholics. In Burtle, V. (Ed.): *Women Who Drink: Alcoholic Experience and Psychotherapy.* Springfield: Charles C Thomas, 1979, pp. 26-48.

Goodwin, D.W.: *Is Alcoholism Hereditary?* Oxford: Oxford University Press, 1976.

Goodwin, D.W., Schulsinger, F., Møller, N., and Hermansen, L. Alcohol problems in adoptees raised apart from alcoholic biological parents. *Arch. Gen. Psychiat. 28:* 238-243, 1973.

Goodwin, D.W., Møller, N., Hermansen, L., Winokur, G., and Guze, S.B.: Drinking problems in adopted and non-adopted sons of alcoholics. *Arch. Gen. Psychiat. 31:* 164-169.

Gorenstein, E.E. Relationships of subclinical depression, psychopathy, and hysteria to patterns of alcohol consumption and abuse in males and females. In Galanter, M. (Ed.): *Currents in Alcoholism. Vol. VII. Recent Advances in Research and Treatment.* New York: Grune and Stratton, 1980, pp. 207-217.

Harbison, R.D., and Evans, M.A.: Teratogenic effects of drug abuse in pregnancy. In Rementería, J.L. (Ed.): *Drug Abuse in Pregnancy and Neonatal Effects.* Saint Louis: C.V. Mosby, 1977, pp. 181-194.

Henderson, G.I., Hoyumpa, A.M., Rothschild, M.A., and Schenker, S.: Effect of ethanol and ethanol-induced hypothermia on protein synthesis in pregnant and fetal rats. *Alcohol Clin. Exp. Res. 4:* 165-177, 1980.

Hirst, M., Evans, D.R., and Gowdey, C.W.: Salsolinol in urine of social drinkers. In Collins, M.A. (Ed.): *Aldehyde Adducts in Alcoholism.* New York: Alan R. Liss, 1985, pp. 85-100.

Hoffman, H., and Jackson, D.N.: Differential personality inventory for male and female alcoholics. *Psychol. Repts. 34:* 21-22, 1974.

Jacobson, G.R.: An introduction to psychological factors in the etiology and treatment of alcoholism. In Galanter, M. (Ed.): *Currents in Alcoholism. Vol. VII. Recent Advances in Research and Treatment.* New York: Grune and Stratton, 1980, pp. 189-205.

Jones, K.L., and Smith, D.W.: Recognition of the fetal alcohol syndrome in early infancy. *Lancet ii:* 99-101, 1973.

Jones, K.L., and Smith, D.W.: The fetal alcohol syndrome. *Teratology 12:* 1-10, 1975.

Kaij, L.: *Alcoholism in Twins: Studies on the Etiology and Sequels of Abuse of Alcohol.* Stockholm: Almqvist and Wiksell, 1960.

Kinsey, B.A.: *The Female Alcoholic: A Social Psychological Study.* Springfield: Charles C Thomas, 1966.

Kolata, G. Fetal alcohol advisory debate. *Science 214:* 642-643, 1981.

Lieber, C.S.: *Medical Disorders of Alcoholism: Pathogenesis and Treatment. Vol. XXII. Major Problems in Internal Medicine.* Philadelphia: W.B. Saunder, 1982.

Light, W.J.H.: *Alcoholism: Its Natural History, Chemistry and General Metabolism.* Springfield: Charles C Thomas, 1985.

Light, W.J.H.: *Neurobiology of Alcohol Abuse.* Springfield: Charles C Thomas, 1986a.

Light, W.J.H.: *Psychodynamics of Alcoholism: A Current Synthesis.* Springfield: Charles C Thomas, 1986b.

Lisansky, E.S.: Alcoholism in women: social and psychological concomitants. *Quart. Journ. Studies on Alcohol 18:* 588-623, 1957.

MacLennan, A. (Ed.): *Women: Their Use of Alcohol and Other Legal Drugs.* Toronto: Addiction Research Foundation of Ontario, 1976.

Mednik, S., Gabrielli, W.F., Jr., and Hutchings, B.: Genetic influences in criminal convictions: evidence from an adoption cohort. *Science: 224:* 891-893.

Melchior, C.L.: Long-lasting effects of tetrahysroisoquinolines. In Sandler, M. (Ed.): *Psychopharmacology of Alcohol.* New York: Raven Press, 1980, pp. 149-153.

Melchior, C.L., and Myers R.D.: Genetic differences in ethanol drinking of the rat following injection of 6-OHDA, 5,6-DHT or 5,7-DHT into the cerebral ventricles. *Pharmac. Biochem. and Behavior 5:* 63-72, 1976.

Melchior, C.L., and Myers, R.D.: Preference for alcohol evoked by tetrahydropapaveroline (THP) chronically infused in the cerebral ventricle of the rat. *Pharmacol. Biochem. and Behavior 7:* 19-35.

Mendelson, R.A., and Huber, A.M.: The effect of ethanol consumption on trace elements in the fetal rat. In Galanter, M. (Ed.): *Currents in Alcoholism: Vol. VII. Recent Advances in Research and Treatment.* New York: Grune and Stratton, 1980.

Mendelson, J.H., and Mello, N.K.: Biological concomitants of alcoholism. *New Engl. Jour. Medicine 301:* 912-921, 1979.

Milam, J.R., and Ketcham, K.: *Under the Influence: A Guide to the Myths and Realities of Alcoholism.* Seattle: Madrona Publishers, 1981.

Mogar, R.F., Wilson, W.M., and Helm, S.T.: Personality subtypes of male and female alcoholic patients. *Internat. Journ. of the Addictions 5:* 99-113.

Moore, K.L. *The Developing Human: Clinically Oriented Embryology,* Second Edition. Philadelphia: W.B. Saunders, 1977.

Morrissey, E.R., and Schuckit, M.A.: Drinking patterns and alcohol-related problems in a population of alcohol detoxification patients: a comparison of males and females. In Galanter, M. (Ed.): *Currents in Alcoholism. Vol. VII. Recent Advances in Research and Treatment.* New York: Grune and Stratton, 1980, pp. 465-480.

Mukherjee, A.B., and Hodgen, G.D.: Maternal ethanol exposure induces transient impairment of umbilical circulation and fetal hypoxia in monkeys. *Science 218:* 700-702, 1982.

Myers, R.D.: Psychopharmacology of alcohol. *Ann. Rev. Pharmacol. Toxicol. 18:* 125-144, 1978.

Myers, R.D.: Multiple metabolite theory, alcohol drinking and the alcogene. In Collins, M.A. (Ed.): *Aldehyde Adducts in Alcoholism.* New York: Alan R. Liss, 1985, pp. 201-220.

Myers, R.D., and Critcher, E.C.: Naloxone alters alcohol drinking induced in the rat by tetrahydropapaveroline (THP) infused ICV. *Pharmacol. Biochem. & Behavior 16:* 827-836, 1982.

Myers, R.D., and Melchior, C.L.: Alcohol drinking: abnormal intake caused by tetrahydropapaveroline in brain. *Science 196:* 554-556, 1977.

Partanen, J., Brunn, K., and Markkanen, T.: *Inheritance of Drinking Behavior.* Helsinki: Finnish Foundation for Alcohol Studies, 1966.

Peele, S.: *How Much is Too Much?* Englewood Cliff: Prentice-Hall, 1981.

Petrie, A.: *Individuality in Pain and Suffering.* Chicago: University of Chicago Press, 1978.

Porjesz, B., and Begleiter, H.: Human brain physiology and alcoholism. In Tarter, R., and van Thiel, D. (Eds.): *Alcohol and the Brain.* New York: Plenum, 1985.

Pratt, O.E.: The fetal alcohol syndrome: transport of nutrients and transfer of alcohol and acetaldehyde from mother to fetus. In Sandler, M. (Ed.): *Psychopharmacology of Alcohol.* New York: Raven Press, 1980.

Richman, S.A., Teichman, M., and Fine, E.W.: Psychosocial differences between male and female alcoholics. In Galanter, M. (Ed.): *Currents in Alcoholism. Vol. VII. Recent Advances in Research and Treatment.* New York: Grune and Stratton, 1980.

Roe, A., and Burks, B.: Adult adjustment of foster children of alcoholic and psychotic parentage and the influence of the foster home. *Memoirs of the Section on Alcohol Studies,*

No. 3. New Haven: Yale University, 1945.

Rosett, H.L.: Clinical pharmacology of the fetal alcohol syndrome. In Majchrowicz, E., and Noble, E.P. (Eds.): *Biochemistry and Pharmacology of Ethanol.* Vol. 2. New York: Plenum Press, 1979.

Rosett, H.L.: The effects of alcohol on the fetus and offspring. In Kalant, O.J. (Ed.): *Alcohol and Drug Problems in Women.* Vol. 5. New York: Plenum Press, 1980, pp. 595-652.

Sandmaier, M.: *The Invisible Alcoholics: Women and Alcohol Abuse in America.* New York: McGraw-Hill, 1980.

Saunders, B.: Psychological aspects of women and alcohol. In Camberwell Council on Alcoholism: *Women and Alcohol.* London and New York: Tavistock Publications, 1980.

Schuckit, M.A., Goodwin, D.W., and Winokur, G.: A study of alcoholism in half siblings. *Amer. Jour. Psychiat. 128:* 122-126, 1972.

Sjöquist, B.: On the origin of salsolinol and 1-carboxysalsolinol. In Collins, M.A. (Ed.): *Aldehyde Adducts in Alcoholism.* New York: Alan R. Liss, 1985, pp. 115-124.

Sjöquist, B.S., Borg, S., and Kvande, H.: Catecholamine derived compounds in urine and cerebrospinal fluid from alcoholics during and after long-standing intoxication. *Subst. Alcohol Act./Misuse 2:* 63-72, 1981.

Sjöquist, B.S., Liljequist, S., and Engel, J.: Increased salsolinol levels in rat striatum and limbic forebrain following chronic ethanol treatment. *Jour. Neurochem. 39:* 259-262, 1982.

Smythe, G.A., and Duncan, M.W.: Precise GC/MS assays for salsolinol and tetrahydropapaveroline: the question of artifacts and dietary sources and the influence of alcohol. *Aldehyde Adducts in Alcoholism.* New York: Liss, 1985, pp. 77-84.

Streissguth, A.P., Landesman-Dwyer, S., Martin, J.C., and Smith, D.W.: Teratogenic effects of alcohol in humans and laboratory animals. *Science 209:* 353-361, 1980.

Sulik, K.K., Johnston, M.C., and Webbs, M.A.: Fetal alcohol syndrome: embryogenesis in a mouse model. *Science 214:* 939-938, 1981.

Summers, M.C.: In Collins, M.A. (Ed.): *Aldehyde Adducts in Alcoholism.* New York: Alan R. Liss, 1985, pp. 39-49.

Synapin, P.J., and Noble, E.P.: Studies in ethanol's effects on cells in culture. In Majchrowicz, E., and Noble, E.P., (Eds.): *Biochemistry and Pharmacology of Ethanol.* Vol. 1. New York: Plenum Press, 1979, pp. 521-540.

Tottmar, O.: In Collins, M.A. (Ed.): *Aldehyde Adducts in Alcoholism.* New York: Alan R. Liss, 1985, pp. 51-56.

Tsuang, M.T., and Vandermy, R.: *Genes and the Mind: Inheritance of Mental Illness.* New York and Oxford: Oxford University Press, 1980.

Vaillant, G.E.: *The Natural History of Alcoholism.* Cambridge: Harvard University Press, 1983.

Vogel, F., and Motulsky, A.G.: *Human Genetics: Problems and Approaches.* Berlin: Springer-Verlag, 1979.

Wartburg, J.P. von. *Acetaldehyde.* In Sandler, M. (Ed.): *Psychopharmacology of Alcohol.* New York: Raven Press, 1980.

INDEX

E

N

O

P